PENGUIN BOOKS

CLIVE

David Snodin is a writer and producer of television drama,
currently based at the BBC. His first play as producer was Clive
Jermain's *The Best Years of Your Life.* His productions since
have included the films *Will You Love Me Tomorrow?* (which he
also co-wrote) and *Lily My Love,* the play *The Interrogation of
John* and a three-part film serial, *Take Me Home,* shown on
BBC1 in May 1989. He has written plays for the theatre and
television and a book called *A Mighty Ferment: Britain in the
Age of Revolution.* For many years he was a script editor at the
BBC, working on classic serials as well as new plays and on the
Shakespeare cycle produced by Jonathan Miller. He was born
in Sweden, spent a good deal of his childhood and youth
abroad, went to Trinity College, Oxford, was a fellow of
Brasenose College, Oxford, and lives in Highgate in North
London.

GW00696855

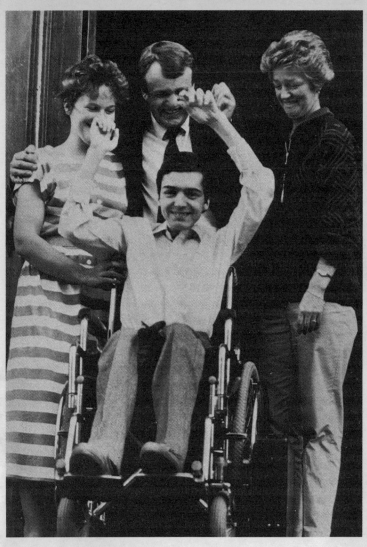

Clive on the steps of the Royal Marsden Hospital, September 1987, with left to right: his friend Fiona Gardner, Gareth Pyne-James, founder of Search '88, and Clive's mother, Maureen. (Press Association)

David Snodin

CLIVE

A BRIEF LIFE

PENGUIN BOOKS

PENGUIN BOOKS

Published by the Penguin Group
Penguin Books Ltd, 27 Wrights Lane, London W8 5TZ, England
Viking Penguin, a division of Penguin Books USA Inc.,
375 Hudson Street, New York, New York 10014, USA
Penguin Books Australia Ltd, Ringwood, Victoria, Australia
Penguin Books Canada Ltd, 2801 John Street, Markham, Ontario, Canada L3R 1B4
Penguin Books (NZ) Ltd, 182–190 Wairau Road, Auckland 10, New Zealand

Penguin Books Ltd, Registered Offices: Harmondsworth, Middlesex, England

First published by Viking 1989
Published in Penguin Books 1990
1 3 5 7 9 10 8 6 4 2

For Clive, of course

CONTENTS

Clive's favourite poem, which he knew by heart, was the following sonnet by Keats:

When I have fears that I may cease to be,
  Before my pen has glean'd my teeming brain,
Before high piléd Books in charactery
  Hold like rich garners the full ripen'd grain –
When I behold upon the night's starr'd face
  Huge cloudy symbols of a high romance,
And feel that I may never live to trace
  Their shadows with the magic hand of Chance:
And when I feel, fair creature of an hour,
  That I shall never look upon thee more,
Never have relish in the faery power
  Of unreflecting Love: then on the shore
    Of the wide world I stand alone and think,
    Till Love and Fame to Nothingness do sink.

FOREWORD

O<small>N</small> a night in September 1987, at about a quarter to midnight, I received a telephone call from BBC *Breakfast Time* asking if I would be prepared to appear on the programme the following morning in order to talk about Clive Jermain, who was, it was generally presumed, going to die at any moment. He was in the Royal Marsden Hospital in the Fulham Road, the country's leading cancer hospital, for the most part unconscious and iller than he had ever been before. If he did die, I would be telephoned again and a car would arrive at six o'clock in the morning to take me to the *Breakfast Time* studio. If, as then seemed unlikely, he survived the night, I would not be disturbed. Of course I could not sleep. I was expecting my telephone to ring again, at whatever hour, and if it did, I would have to be awake again soon enough. So I spent those sleepless hours writing about Clive. 'I first met Clive Jermain in January 1985 . . .' I began. I described how and why we had met, what he had meant to me, what I thought of him, why I considered him extraordinary, exemplary, humbling (and sometimes infuriating), and how very wretched I felt about the fact that he was going to die, even though his death had been anticipated for so long. I wrote about twenty packed pages and much of what I wrote has gone into this book. I understood while I was writing that I was putting it all down not just for my sake, and to fill a few sleepless hours, but because of a need to impart this sad but courageous twenty-two-year-old's singularity to others.

Clive did not die that night, or the next, or the next (it was touch and go for about a week), or indeed for another six months.

11

His remission received substantial publicity (of the 'cancer-beating hero' kind), and because of this, allied to the fact that his play *The Best Years of Your Life* had been repeated on television in tandem with a documentary about him as he lay semi-comatose in hospital, I was contacted by two editors at Viking Penguin, Pamela Dix and Geraldine Cook, who commissioned me to write a book *with* Clive about his life. It would not be a ghosted autobiography, because I wanted to play a greater part in it than that and felt that an essential aspect of Clive's story was the effect he had on those who knew him; but much of the book would nonetheless be in Clive's own words. Always eager for a memorial, Clive, though weak, was immediately and enthusiastically receptive to the idea of writing about himself, his achievements and his situation with my help.

From the very first he was determined that we should together paint a truthful portrait, pulling no punches. He wanted no glossing or fabrication for the sake of painless reading, and held no brief for hyperbole or blinkered adulation. He was proud of what he had achieved in his short life, for he understood better than anyone what the odds had been against his achieving anything at all in the circumstances, but he now wanted to convey (with increasing and touching insistence the closer he came to death) those very odds rather than the achievements. He told me how a friend who had visited him on one of his 'toilet days', and who had seen him on television only a short while previously, had pointed out the contrast she immediately noted between the assured young presenter she had seen on the screen and the very ill and incapacitated young man lying before her at that moment, and she had said, 'If only they knew.' So in those last few months of Clive's life we talked mainly of the more troubled aspects of his existence – the great sickness, the unimaginable pain, the frustration and occasional despair caused by his disability, and his thoughts on death, of which he had once been very afraid. These were the things he now wanted others to 'know about'. Clive always grimaced when words like 'heroic', 'courageous', 'miraculous', 'fearless' and 'brave' were used to describe him. He knew that if the dark side of his story was told, the unarguable courage and manifold achievements would in a sense look after themselves in the narrative, and I very much hope they have done.

Neither of us had any idea how this 'book' that we were supposed to be writing together would turn out. Clive himself could actually 'write' nothing now. At the best of times he had found the physical business of writing very hard, even when he was feeling clear and creative, but now he was suffering from overwhelming bouts of exhaustion and the will to create had gone. He could talk, though, with characteristic eloquence and frankness (and humour), and so we talked, for many hours over the months, with a little tape recorder beside us. We decided that others would have to contribute to the story – those nearest to Clive, primarily, his family and close friends. 'You'll have to ask Maureen that,' he would say, or 'Elaine's got a few good things to say about me.' But a sense of time running out made me concentrate on conversing with Clive while he was still alive. Each conversation could so well have been the last, and there was always more to learn and be moved by.

Then he died. Some days before his death he gave me a thick sheaf of papers, disorganized but mesmerizing, many of them heartbreaking, which were what he liked to call his 'thoughts'. With these, the many tapes, and several boxes of scripts, roughly typed ideas, scenarios and letters lent to me by Clive's mother, I had to set about continuing the book on my own. In my sadness I wrote about Clive's funeral during the course of the weekend after it occurred. But there was a terrible hiatus in my efforts when I realized that I had made a close and quite exceptional friend whom I would now never see again, and I could not write a word. Then I started to record conversations with those 'others' whom Clive had said I should speak to. It is a reflection of their own considerable courage that they did not allow their own deep grief to get in the way of their honesty. They knew too that it was the truth that mattered, not the gloss. Once I felt that I had enough material the book proved to be remarkably easy to write, because of the simple strength of the tale that had to be told, and because I was driven even more fervently by that 'need to impart' that I had felt the previous September when I thought Clive was going to die.

When the close ones whom I have quoted at length and often in the ensuing pages – Clive's mother Maureen, his brother Lee, his best friend Elaine, and Fiona, his nurse for a time at the Royal Marsden – read the first draft of the book, they were not disappointed or appalled but they were somewhat (though amicably) disturbed, and had the honesty to tell me so. They could not, and did not wish to, deny the truth of what I had written (except in the case of a few small details of fact, which have been duly corrected), but overall they felt that the story I had told was perhaps too bleak to be *entirely* fair to Clive's memory. I had not, they said, written enough about the 'good times', of which there were many, or the laughter, of which there was an abundance, in spite of the pain and the affliction. I have tried to shift the story's emphasis a little in places to accommodate the views of those nearest to Clive, acknowledging that at times I have emphasized the dark side at the expense of the many lighter moments. In general, though, I stand by what I have written. I have tried to depict, in clear and often painful detail, the wretched and debilitating circumstances under which Clive had to struggle so hard to achieve what he did achieve, and to make space in a life of anxiety and agony for those many 'good times' and for that copious and infectious laughter. And, as I have already said, Clive's wish was that the book should carry such an emphasis. I hope above all that this story as it is told in the pages that follow is a reasonably adequate and fair response to the words of the friend of Clive's who said, 'If only they knew . . .'

It is to Clive's mother, Maureen Jermain, that I owe my most profound thanks, for helping me to record her son's life and spirit by being so very friendly, open, patient, honest and brave during what inevitably was still a time of deep grief. I am also grateful to her for allowing me to become her friend. Clive's good friend Elaine Chanter and his brother Lee Jermain possessed similarly exceptional courage in recollection, for they both, like Maureen, still miss him dreadfully. I am enormously indebted to the two of them. Fiona Gardner, who also grieves, gave me her time with great fortitude and truthfulness, and I am deeply thankful to her.

Others I wish to thank are Dick Sharples and Anthony Parker, two of Clive's 'friends and advisers', Chris Hutchins, the producer of *One in Four*, Stephen Kramer, one of Clive's carers, and Peter Wells, whose eloquent and perceptive insights into the nature of

FOREWORD

Clive's faith helped me write the last pages of this story. The newsreader Martyn Lewis took time off in a busy schedule to talk about what he remembered of Clive, as did Dr Geoff Hanks of the Royal Marsden Hospital, who also checked the medical history in the typescript. Others who read the first draft, who did not know Clive but for whose comments and suggestions I am grateful, are my friend Susan Marling and my mother and father. Adrian Shergold and Maria Hannon kindly allowed me to look at and use the transcripts of many hours of conversations with Clive for the documentary about him which they co-directed. Pamela Dix and Geraldine Cook of Viking Penguin displayed exceptional patience and understanding as they waited for me to come up with something.

Finally I want to thank Clive himself, for the fact of having given me the privilege of knowing him, for his own enormous courage in talking and remembering when he was so very ill, for entrusting me with the task of writing this book, and for providing me with the most moving year of *my* life. It is to his memory, of course, that this book is dedicated. I hope he feels I have acquitted myself well. He will know, I trust, that the pages that follow, whatever their faults and omissions, were written out of deep love.

Highgate, September 1988

1

DEATH

I was in Clive's sitting-room on a Wednesday afternoon in February waiting, I presumed, for him to die. With me was Clive's younger brother Lee, who was looking flushed with understandable excitement because he had just bought himself his first car – a very shiny blue six-year-old Ford Fiesta Ghia. Earlier that afternoon I had been with him and his mother to pick it up, and he had taken us on a bit of a squeal round the estate in Peckham in which Clive lived. As we waited in the sitting-room, we talked cars and engine capacities and insurance. The television was on, as it always was, flickering soundless pictures. Clive's mother Maureen came in. 'He's fighting for his breath in there, and here am I dying for a fag.' She lit up. 'He's never been this bad,' she said. It had been decided that Clive's state was serious enough to warrant another visit from the doctor, but he was on 'the other side of town' and would not arrive for another hour at least. Clive had developed a chest infection which was producing so much phlegm that the fear was that he would choke to death. It was a possibility that Clive himself found more frightening than any other.

As was always the case at Clive's place, others started to arrive – those closest to him now, because of his state. There were few casual visitors at this stage. Elaine arrived first. She worked in the local baker's, was twenty-four, and had known Clive since she was fourteen and he was twelve. Then came Fiona, a nurse from the Royal Marsden Hospital who had become a loyal friend, and her husband Craig. Fiona was heavily pregnant. I was the comparative stranger in this group of close ones. They did not sit in awed silence because of the situation, but were capable of loud small-talk and even laughter, although I did think that Maureen was looking unspeakably tired.

I started to make movements to leave. 'You'll say goodbye to Clive, won't you?' said Maureen, and with her I went in to see him. He was lying on his back, his mouth wide open, ashen as he had been for many months now, taking deep rasping breaths. The only acknowledgement of our presence was a brief flicker of closed eyelids. I sat on one side of the bed, Maureen on the other. I could say very little. I offered the merely trite, muttering a few pleasantries, passing on the best wishes of mutual friends, but for the most part I just sat there, and Maureen did too, speaking only rarely, looking down at her son, now and then letting quiet tears get the better of her. I found myself, since verbal contact seemed so inadequate, holding his hand, squeezing it sometimes, stroking its extraordinary smallness with my forefinger, in a fumbling attempt to convey sympathy, sorrow, anger, love. I had intended to say a quick goodbye and leave, but I was there for well over an hour.

With time, the breathing seemed to become less difficult, and there was relief all round. Clive began to respond to being addressed, and took a little drink to slake his parched lips and throat. Elaine, who could always make him laugh, cracked a joke and he smiled weakly. The doctor arrived, and there was the usual hush in the presence of medical authority. I decided it was time to go. I said goodbye to Clive and added, only naturally, that I would see him soon. Although I had known all afternoon that I had been in the presence of imminent death, I did not assume at the moment of saying goodbye that I would never see this exceptional young man again.

I telephoned Clive's flat on the Sunday following my visit. Maureen answered. 'Oh, he's quite chirpy today,' she said, almost as surprised in her tone as I was in my reaction. 'He wants to get up. We've been going through more of his papers, his school reports – we've been laughing at those.' Clive was asleep when I called, so I did not speak to him. I fully expected to see him some time during the ensuing week.

On the Tuesday, which was 1 March 1988, St David's Day, I

returned from the cinema and a meal and there was one crackly message on my answering machine: 'It's Fiona. Clive died tonight at nine o'clock. It was very peaceful. I'll talk to you soon.' Later, mercifully (What do you do? I wanted to ring, I felt I couldn't), Fiona rang again. It was at one o'clock in the morning. I had sat for two hours, sleepless and impotent. She reiterated that Clive had died peacefully, and added that he had been in the company of the four people closest to him – his mother, his brother Lee, his best friend Elaine, and Fiona – and that, more importantly than anything else, he had died at home. There had been no pain. He had simply had a blackout. I said to Fiona: 'Tell Maureen my thoughts are with her and if she wants me to do anything, anything . . .'

The uncertainty of cancer is its greatest inclemency. It can sometimes appear to inflict more cruelty upon those who witness it than it most undoubtedly does upon those who have it. Those closest to Clive had lived with an appalling and exhausting uncertainty, without let-up, for many months prior to the time in February when I last saw him. Of course he had been punishingly ill for years, and had nearly died one or two times since his cancer was first diagnosed, but never before those final months had there been such a relentless possibility of death at any moment. All in all that last half year, with its ups and downs, its sharp moments of panic and relief, its sleepless nights, and the simple and terrible fatigue of waiting for death, had constituted a pitiless battering on the hearts and minds of those immediately involved in the whole merciless process. This is not to imply that all was misery even now. There was laughter, as there always had been, much to remember with a smile, and a good party or two.

The slow baleful slide towards inevitable death had started towards the end of the previous August. Clive was rushed to the Royal Marsden Hospital in the Fulham Road, in extreme pain. The tumour at the top of his spine was attacking the brain stem with apparently irreversible finality. His mother was on holiday in the Canary Islands at the time, but Elaine was with him. She remembered: 'He was wrapped up in his red blanket, and he was saying, "Please don't leave me, I'm so scared, please don't leave me," I said, "I won't." And he was screaming with this pain in his head, holding my hand, and I said, "I promise I won't leave you," and all I could think of was "This is it. This must be it."'

She was told by the doctor who had supervised the control of Clive's pain for some years that Clive would be 'lucky if he made it through the night'. Elaine then had to try to get hold of his mother – she had no address, but contact was made through the British Consulate in Tenerife. 'I didn't know Maureen very well then,' she recalled, 'but I cried down the phone. I said, "Please come back." She said, "I'm on my way."'

Maureen could not get a flight until the following evening, though, so Elaine was with Clive while he slipped in and out of a comatose state for almost twenty-four hours before his mother arrived. His favourite nurse Fiona was also there, and later in the day Peter Wells, a priest with whom he had become friendly and for whose presence he had specifically asked, sat by his bed and said a few prayers with him, and they read a few of Clive's favourite psalms together. Again Elaine thought that Clive was going to die before seeing his mother: 'He was so weak, and he said, "Please tell her I can't hold on any more, I want to go now, I've had enough of fighting the pain," and I said, "She'll understand, Clive."'

When Maureen turned up at last, having been flown by helicopter from Luton Airport thanks to the offices of the cancer charity Search 88, with which Clive had strong associations, the weak young man said to his mother, "What are you doing back?" and his mother replied, "It was too hot out there, Clive." Lee remembered that when *he* arrived at Clive's bedside, three days after his mother, the first thing Clive asked him was, "Was it hot out there?"

By uncomfortable coincidence, Clive's television play *The Best Years of Your Life* had been scheduled to be broadcast a second time as he lay semi-comatose in his hospital bed. A documentary about him was to be shown the night after the repeat of the play. Both transmissions had to await Clive's mother's permission before they could be given the go-ahead at such a critical time, but Maureen was not slow to agree to their being shown. 'He'd want it,' she said.

DEATH

As the producer of the play, I had to remain in continual contact with the hospital in case Clive died and an announcement had to be made on television either before or after the play or documentary. I visited Clive in hospital the day after the play had been shown. He had already survived three nights longer than had been at first expected. Nevertheless, he still appeared unconscious when I arrived and looked as close to death as I imagined it was possible to look. In the years I had known him I had seen him look very ill but never as gruesomely ill as this. To be frank, I felt shocked and sickened, and for the first time in a sheltered life – understanding at that instant how sheltered it had been – I realized clearly the ghastly indignity of cancer. I felt ashamed for him. I felt that if he had had any control over his state he would have asked me to leave for a time while he composed himself to receive me more decorously. Whenever he was visited Clive had always wanted to 'look his best'. Many were the times that I had had to wait in his sitting-room, sometimes for a good half hour, while he had 'prepared himself' to receive me. It was an entirely pardonable vain streak in his nature. He could be very ashamed of his disability, unable to free himself wholly from the concept of his condition as something of a stigma. Now he looked worse than I had ever seen him and I wanted not to look at him, because of my squeamishness and also a degree of shame on his behalf. His skin was grey, the enormous rings under his eyes were truly black, his hair was matted with sweat, his mouth was gaping, although sometimes he would close it and swallow in order to try to relieve the dryness, and his lips had to be continually swabbed.

Maureen, looking deathly herself from lack of sleep, told me to say something to him ('Talk to him, David, he can hear you') but I remained haplessly silent. Fiona came in to tell Maureen that it was time to turn Clive over and this they then did, the two of them, pulling back the covers of the bed and revealing Clive's naked, pale and shrivelled body, his legs and arms mere sticks. I suspected again that Clive, had he been able to dictate the situation, would far rather I had not been present, but Maureen and Fiona performed the task so quickly and efficiently that I did not have time to turn away, let alone leave, and no doubt as far as they were concerned this was not the time for prurience or excessive propriety.

In time Clive gained greater consciousness of what was happening and of who was in his small darkened hospital room, and we began to have a faltering conversation, Clive speaking in a hoarse and often barely audible whisper. He seemed very drugged. His voice strengthened after a while, and he asked everyone who was in the room then to leave the two of us alone for a few minutes. I knew at once that he was going to say goodbye to me. He did not say it straight out, as a direct 'goodbye'. After a few minutes of trivial exchanging of information he started to thank me, for getting his play made, for having faith in him, and he said he was sorry that he had not managed to write a second play as he so wanted to. Then he said, openly and without preamble, that he loved me, that he was so full of love. I replied with the tears welling that I loved him too, very much. It was an extraordinary moment – the most moving of my life. And then I really did think that that was the last I would see of him.

But he slowly improved, and on subsequent evenings he was visited by celebrities – Terry Wogan, upon whose show he had appeared only a few weeks previously, and the television newsreader Martyn Lewis, who remembered that from being semicomatose and apparently unaware of those around him, Clive became suddenly voluble and alert, asking detailed and precise questions about the finer points of newsreading, about the positions of cameras, the use of the teleprompter, the handling of late items. Martyn Lewis also recalled that when Clive expressed a sudden and specific wish for 'a bar of Galaxy milk chocolate', he felt duty bound to go out into the cold night and search high and low for a late night shop that sold them.

Wogan was apparently treated not unlike visiting royalty. In spite of the appalling state of his health, Clive tried to behave with dignity and with as much normality as possible. He insisted on sitting up, and asked the famous man if he would like tea or coffee. When Wogan said coffee, Clive turned to Elaine and said peremptorily, 'Elaine. Coffee.' Wogan asked Elaine: 'Does he always boss you about like that?'

*

Clive did not of course die that September. Fiona told me how she had had to leave him for a few days in hospital, convinced – as I had been that time I saw him – that she would never see him again: 'I'd been staying up at the hospital with him for about a week, ten days, and Maureen had come back and we were all up there with Elaine, and Lee, and I had to go up to Yorkshire, it was Craig's parents' fortieth wedding anniversary, and Clive was really quite bad and I didn't want to go, and I felt very torn, and I sat and spent a long time with Clive and we were chatting about this and he knew I was going up and he said, "Don't be sad, I won't be here when you come back, but I'm happy and I'll always be with you," and we talked about a lot of things, so . . . fully expecting to hear within the next twenty-four hours that he'd died, off I went. I only actually stayed in Yorkshire for about fifteen hours; we came back and I went up to the ward and I saw Clive's chair outside his room, and I thought, "That's it," and I remember all the pillows were on the chair, so I went into the office and tried to prepare myself and they said, "Oh, Clive's all right, he's sitting up in bed," and I thought, "Shit," and I went into his room and he was sitting there smiling and he said . . . "I really thought I was going and I haven't."'

Some days after this, Clive was photographed on the steps of the Royal Marsden, his usable hand raised in triumph, by the assembled press. A press release announced 'CANCER FIGHTER CLIVE CONFOUNDS DOCTORS', and quoted a Search 88 worker as saying that 'His favourite pastime is confounding the doctors and he has done it again, although he is still very weak. Work has been piling up on his desk here so I'm sure he will want to get back in as soon as possible.' A spokesman for the Royal Marsden said: 'Clive's condition has improved remarkably . . . It is great news and it shows a tremendous fighting spirit.' The newspapers brayed: 'FERGIE CANCER HERO COMES BACK FROM THE DEAD,' 'THE CANCER VICTIM WHO REFUSED TO DIE,' '"FERGIE IS MY HERO," SAYS MR MIRACLE.'

The 'Fergie' connection was based on the fact that the Duchess of York was the official patron of Search 88. Although she had indeed sent a message of support to Clive at the hospital, she had not, as the papers liked to convey, 'phoned him every day'. But Clive, who himself had an instinctive understanding of a good story, gamely responded to the 'Fergie' questions: 'It's all thanks to Fergie . . . it was a big morale boost knowing the Duchess was cheering for me.' But this particular story ended with Clive's true priorities: 'God decided it wasn't my time. And what helped keep me going was the support of my family, particularly my mum.' If the 'Fergie' quotes were not wholly truthful, the last one undoubtedly was.

Clive was never to return in any way to the state of health that he had been in before the coma. He had to be watched with a vigilance he had not known previously. He had blackouts, always as a result of being moved into an upright position too rapidly. He had to be careful when rising in the mornings. He tried to continue his association with Search 88, although his interest in the charity had weakened considerably. He was now more dedicated to his job as a co-presenter on a BBC Television programme on disability called *One in Four*, and with rehearsals for a stage version of his television play at a fringe theatre in the King's Road. He also began a series of detailed conversations with me for this book.

In November, however, he was back in hospital, and once again the outlook was dark. This time round, the primary fear of his relatives and friends was not so much the possibility of death as the danger that whatever time that was left to him, short or long, would be spent as a helpless 'vegetable', or at best as a total stranger to them. Elaine had been telephoned by Clive's carer, who told her that Clive had been blacked out for an hour. When Elaine turned up at the flat, 'He was lying on his back having a fit.' He was in a state of semi-conscious burbling incoherence, his tongue rolling around uncontrollably inside his mouth. 'I said to the carer why's he on his back, and the first thing I did was pulled him into a sitting position and grabbed his tongue so he wouldn't choke.'

She telephoned for an ambulance, then rang Clive's doctor, and then Maureen. The doctor was understandably livid when he was told how long Clive had been in the state he was in. Maureen arrived just as Clive was being carried to the ambulance.

'He was lying there,' said Maureen, 'gurgling and screaming.'
She was more frightened for her son than she had ever been. 'I
said to the doctor that night, I can cope with anything but I don't
think I can cope with seeing Clive becoming silly.'

When I [...] or three days after this admission –
[...] of the stage version of his play –
[...] o make some kind of sense, but
t[...] s train of thought, in that phrases
a[...] up that seemed to spring from
no[...] ot unlike senility. Maureen recall[...] me questions – 'What day is it?'
and [...] ally, at half-hourly intervals. I
notic[...] e ward's day-room, along with
severa[...] of what he said seemed to be
quite [...] l suddenly say, 'What do you
know, [...] e had a wild and largely un-
recogniz[...] ld also tut-tut consistently, a
manneris[...] fore, but which now seemed
more insis[...]

Whatev[...] our, whether it was the effect
on his brai[...] ugs he was on, or a mixture
of both, it was very disturbing indeed. It was all too easy to
comprehend Maureen's simple terror. As I was about to go home,
Clive said something to me that in the circumstances had a frightening clarity. He said quietly, 'This is serious, believe me,' which
was I presumed another way of telling me that he could die at
any moment and that if he did, then this was another goodbye.
Mercifully, the next day he remembered nothing of my visit, nor
of anyone else who was there, nor indeed of anything that had
happened. It had been a particularly bad day and best forgotten
anyway, but the fact that he could remember nothing of it whatsoever frightened him.

Within a week he was back at home with his thought-patterns
normal again. He saw his play in the theatre at last. He presented
further episodes of *One in Four*. He appeared on a special Christmas
edition of the *Wogan* show. He took part in the *Children in Need*
telethon. But he was weakening all the time. My conversations
with him continued, and I learnt more and more about his life

and thoughts. He became franker, more ready to tell me what he really thought, to detail the true nature of his fears and frustrations, as the weeks passed. But towards the end of January he did not seem to want to say any more. The effort of recollection and speculation was too exhausting. I knew I had to stop asking questions. Watching him die was all I could do. At the start of February he was in hospital again with a bladder infection.

Visiting him, I felt that I had seen him look iller before, but never so very, very sad. He was now well beyond forced composure or vanity, and regardless of who was in the room at the time he would suddenly break into great sobs, and would lie there crying, as one sat and watched, incapable of reassurance. I was reminded of a line in his play: 'What can you say? You can't say everything's going to be all right, can you?' The tears that I saw and sat helplessly before seemed to express an enormous frustration and wordless despair at his incapacity as he lay there so dependent, at his inability to do anything but wait for the end, and perhaps indeed at his inability to hasten his end. For me that terrible weeping seemed to symbolize everything that had been kept in abeyance for the sake of decorum for so long – a great lamentation at the endless pain and heartbreak of it all. I for one had never seen him cry before. 'I feel so good for about two minutes,' he kept saying.

I did not know at that time that he was discovering a certain spiritual contentment and a feeling of completeness during that last stay in the Royal Marsden. He became ready to die. When he felt prepared, he no longer wanted to be in hospital. All he wanted was to go home. As far as he was concerned, nothing more could be done for him, but it was very important to him that he should die at home. In the middle of one night he discharged himself. He was asked to wait at least until daylight but he was insistent. His frustration was increased by the fact that he had to wait for a blood transfusion that to him seemed to take an inordinately and unfairly long time. It was this transfusion that kept Clive alive for another fortnight, but to him it seemed a delaying tactic and part of a general medical conspiracy not to let him have his way. At last, however, his mother drove him back to Peckham, at about one o'clock in the morning.

I visited Clive a few times during his last two weeks, hoping to talk further but soon realizing that his overwhelming concerns lay elsewhere. In the time that was left he had arrangements to make – the personal and emotional tidying-up that ensures what is known as 'a good death', a kind of clearing of the accounts with loved ones. 'He had so much to get done,' said Maureen. 'We were making all these lists, me and Elaine and Fiona. It was "ring this person, ring that person".' Clive also had piles of papers, scribblings, 'thoughts', letters, and a host of photographs that he wanted to sort out. He started to pick out the ones that he thought would be most useful to the book and gave them to me. A good part of the time he dozed, however. He found it hard to sleep at night because of the pain, but was also anxious not to be 'drugged up', as he put it. So, according to Elaine, 'We had to crush up Valium in his ice-cream so he wouldn't notice.' When he did consent to dosages of Valium, to relax him, and diamorphine, to relieve the pain, they had to be administered in suppository form because of his difficulty in swallowing. His chest infection made it very hard for him to breathe as well. He had a 'nebulizer', or breathing apparatus, by his bed continuously. He was frightened more than anything else of choking to death. 'He wasn't afraid of dying,' said Fiona, 'just of the way it might happen.'

To the fear of not being able to breathe must have been added the fear that such a crisis, or another blackout, might have panicked those around him into sending him speedily back to hospital – so he was careful to receive his mother's reassurance that this must on no account happen, that she must be strong in the matter, however much she might be tempted to hand him back to the experts at a desperate moment. She told me this on that February afternoon when I saw him for the last time: 'He's said that he mustn't go back in, *whatever happens.*' This was Maureen's way of telling me that he had come home to die – no one had told me of his wish in so many words – and I understood it as such, but as I have already said, I did not suspect that death would arrive as soon as it did. I was sure that the waiting would drag on for weeks, even months, as it had done until now, and those closer to Clive than I was assumed the same. Death, it seems, can never be entirely expected.

CLIVE: A BRIEF LIFE

'We didn't expect him to die that day,' said Fiona. 'He'd actually been quite well. The first week he was home he was awful. About a week before he died he had a terrible colour, and it looked as if every breath would be his last. We were absolutely positive he was going to go. And the day he died he was really quite happy.' Elaine said: 'It was a shock. I knew he was going to die, but it had just gone on and on, so when it came I wasn't expecting it. And I didn't think he'd go like that. He just went, like that. I thought he'd go into a coma or something.'

Maureen, too, had been prepared for a long vigil. After Clive had come out of hospital for the last time she had told her employers at a department store in North London that she was going to look after her son full-time and she did not know when she would be back: 'When I told them at work that I wasn't coming in any more because I knew Clive hadn't got long to go, I told them I didn't know when I'd be back, because I honestly thought it'd be months, not just two weeks, so it was a shock. I just thought that he'd just get worse and worse and that he would sleep a lot and gradually go into a coma and go that way.' Lee said: 'I really didn't believe it was going to be then, because there'd been so many times when I thought it was going to happen and it hadn't.'

Clive was going to get out of bed that evening and sit up for a proper meal. Maureen had prepared 'stew and dumplings, one of his favourites'. An old friend had come to see him – Claire, a physiotherapist, whom he had not seen for a long time. Because of the danger of blacking out, Clive had to wait in bed, sitting up, for at least half an hour before being lifted out of bed and put into his wheelchair. On this occasion he sat in bed talking and reminiscing quite garrulously with Claire. Maureen recalled a lot of laughter emanating from her son's little back bedroom. Lee too remembered the laughter: 'I came in from work and I could hear them laughing and joking in there.' Clive had always had a tendency to 'hold court' in this room, rather relishing the audiences he held from his semi-prone position, king-like. Fiona put it well: 'You arrive and you're kept waiting for ten or fifteen minutes and you're beginning to think, "Does he want to see me or not?" and you *know* Clive's in there making you wait just that bit

28

longer – I mean there were things he had to do but he did quite enjoy making you wait.' On this occasion Claire was summoned in to see Clive and Fiona remembered him 'sitting there, smiling and charming, quite like his old self'. After talking with Claire for about an hour, at around half past eight, Clive announced that he was hungry and ready to get up. Maureen came into the bedroom to help Claire lift him into his wheelchair.

'He just went,' Elaine recalled. 'He was happy, no pain, nothing, he wanted to get up and have his dinner, dumplings and stew, and he just went, like that.' Maureen said that she 'put his legs over the bed in the usual way and sat him into his chair and his eyes rolled and he went funny and just fell back, immediately'. Lee was called in from the sitting-room and helped Maureen lift Clive back on to the bed. Then Elaine came in, then Fiona. There was no panic because nobody thought to begin with that this was anything but just another blackout; within half an hour or so, as usual, Clive would very probably come round. So they waited.

Fiona was understandably the first to suspect that this was the end: 'He just wasn't responding. He was barely breathing. He was blue. Purple. I just had a gut feeling he wasn't going to come round. If he was going to he should have started to come round but he just didn't.' She felt his pulse, kept talking to him, and repeatedly looked at Maureen, saying, 'I'm not getting anything.' Lee remembered that Fiona asked him to fetch a flannel and a spoon from the kitchen ('That's what she used to hold down Clive's tongue when he was unconscious'), and when he returned, 'I saw that he was blue, mauve, and I'd never seen him like that before, so that was when I knew.' Maureen described what she imagined to be the exact moment of expiration: 'He wasn't breathing but there was just something like one little bit of breath, just one expiring little breath, and that was it.' He had blacked out at half past eight and he died at nine o'clock.

'When I realized he'd died,' said Fiona, 'I turned to Maureen and said, "I think he's gone," and she just kept looking at him, everyone kept looking at him, waiting for him to open his eyes and say, "What are you all staring at?"' Lee recollected a long silence: 'No one said anything. You just don't know what to do, you just stand there, we just stood there . . .'

Maureen asked to be left alone with her son for a while, and she sat with him for about half an hour. Clive was straightened out on the bed. Someone made a cup of coffee. Fiona made telephone calls. Her husband Craig was sent out to buy a bottle of Irish whiskey and two hundred cigarettes. Lee could not recall any tears being shed that night: 'I don't think anyone cried. You can't cry when it happens. You just think, "How can he be dead?"' He was not in the room when Elaine broke down and cried, profusely but briefly. Despite the unexpectedness of the time and manner of Clive's passing, the prevalent feeling, recalled by all those present, was one of calmness. 'After all,' said Fiona, 'we'd all spent the last fortnight with him coming to accept that he was dying, as much as he accepted it and realized it.' Lee remembered how the the presence of death in the flat imposed upon everyone a need to be silent, to tip-toe everywhere, to whisper – 'You felt if you dropped something it'd wake Clive up.'

Maureen sat with Clive all night. Left alone, she wept. Elaine recollected feeling the deepest sense of loss the next morning, when the undertakers came to take Clive away: 'That was the worst, when they actually took him out of the house, that was when I knew he'd gone.' Lee was similarly affected: 'It was horrible. They asked us all to go into the front room, and they shut all the doors, and you saw the coffin go out of the front door. It suddenly made it real. Before that I didn't believe it. When you see the coffin that's when you know.' Elaine was to be even more upset a few days later when she saw Clive laid out in his coffin at the local undertaker's: 'I went to see him at the Chapel of Rest. Maureen said he looked lovely but it shook me badly, seeing him. The only thing that was natural, I thought, was his hair. Nothing else was him. He wasn't my Clive.'

Clive's death made the breakfast television news the following morning, on both channels, and was even announced on the more demure nine o'clock morning news on BBC Radio Four. Maureen was distressed at the immediate assumption on the part of the broadcasters that Clive had died in hospital. Understandably she wanted it to be known that he had ended his life surrounded by his family and loved ones, as he had wished, and at home, as he had wished – perhaps she desired some tacit acknowledgement of her own fortitude in not yielding to the temptation at a time of crisis to send him back into the hands of the doctors. The misapprehension was corrected in later bulletins.

The newspapers did not pick up the story until the following day, and when they did it was of course the royal connection that was emphasized: 'FERGIE'S FRIEND LOSES FIGHT,' 'FERGIE'S CANCER HERO DIES.' The Duchess of York was in Los Angeles at the time and was said to be 'deeply saddened' by the news. 'CANCER HERO CLIVE DIES AMONG HIS ROYAL TREASURES,' announced the *Daily Mail*, reporting that he had 'died surrounded by the people and things he loved most . . . in his bedroom stuffed with precious mementoes including a framed letter signed "Sarah" and an enamel pill-box inscribed "S"'. Maureen was quoted as saying of Clive, 'He was a one-off', which was a succinctly fine way of describing him.

The 'quality' dailies gave him considered tributes. *The Times* wrote that he was 'a self-possessed and fluent young man, whose own condition taught him to talk about bereavement, grief and abandonment with equanimity. In him there appeared to be no self-pity.' The *Independent* wrote of the 'Kafkaesque nightmare' of his life, and Mark Lawson, the television critic, said of Clive's play: 'It needs no allowances from anyone. *The Best Years of Your Life* takes a place alongside *The Diary of Anne Frank* and Christy Nolan's *Under the Eye of the Clock* – other works by old minds in young and threatened bodies – as a vital external expression of a rare interior experience.' When reading this summation I had no doubt that of all the tributes it would have been the one that Clive would have treasured the most.

The funeral was fixed for the Thursday following the week of Clive's death, at eleven o'clock in the morning. He was given quite a send-off, 'Just as he wanted', said Maureen. The press was there, the photographers, and the television cameras. Maureen had permitted their presence because that, too, was what Clive 'would have wanted'. He had said on many occasions, after all, that what had perturbed him most about the death of his grandmother, who had looked after him for a good part of his life and who had died of cancer herself four years before him, was the sad way in which her passing had gone unnoticed by the world: 'I remember turning on the television and there was news from everywhere, and I kept thinking, "They've said nothing about my Nan dying."' Clive was determined that *his* departure should not be ignored. The efforts of the last eight or so years of his life had been channelled into the pursuit of fame largely for that reason. It would also have seemed somewhat unfitting – something would have been missing – if the final laying to rest of this young product of the media age, whose obsession since early childhood had been television and who sought so assiduously to become part of the television phenomenon, had not been a part of that phenomenon itself.

It was a fresh hazy March day. Many friends and a few relatives – Clive did not have many relatives – assembled at Clive's flat prior to joining the cortège to the cemetery. Maureen presided over the proceedings with controlled grace. The pavement in front of the flat was covered with bouquets and wreaths spilling over from the front lawn – a great spread of flowers, with tributes attached. The most striking arrangement was a gigantic floral CLIVE from the local bakery, a hundred yards or so from the flat, where Elaine worked.

Like weddings, funerals can be occasions for gossip and speculation, and Clive's funeral was no exception. The main topic of contemplation, among those who had gathered early enough, concerned the probability or otherwise of Clive's father turning up to pay his last respects to his son. He had not seen Clive for four years, although he lived just round the corner, and he had effectively been separated from Maureen for most of Clive's life, although they were still not divorced. Clive had seemed to sense a slow but immutable loss of interest which, he felt, began soon after his tumour had been diagnosed. He had inflexible feelings towards his father which had understandably influenced his mother's attitude, so it took some staunchness on her part to invite her husband to the funeral as she did, and to allow him, if he so wished, to sit beside her in the cortège. 'He was Clive's dad after all,' she said to me. Conjecture ceased as the father turned up. Few present had seen him before, but everyone had heard of him. Wisely, perhaps, he had brought support – his girlfriend, and his brother and his wife.

DEATH

The cortège began its slow dignified crawl to the cemetery at about a quarter to eleven. There were two hearses, one for the coffin and one to carry all the flowers. The huge floral CLIVE was placed above the windscreen on the first hearse. In the black car behind the hearses sat Clive's father and mother, Elaine, Lee, and Maureen's boyfriend Les. A trail of about ten private cars followed. Stopping the traffic, policemen and policewomen saluted, rigid with respect until we had passed. Old men stood still on the pavement and doffed their hats. 'I don't think they'd seen anything like it round those parts for a long time,' Maureen recalled proudly. With perfect undertaker's timing, we arrived at Honor Oak Cemetery, Camberwell, at eleven o'clock on the dot, turning into the crackling gravelled driveway to see what must have been well over another hundred friends and colleagues waiting.

The coffin was lifted out of the hearse and carried into the chapel, and the congregation filed in behind it, to the accompaniment of a pop song called 'Hold On – Clive's Song', which had been recorded the previous summer for the Search 88 charity. Even judged as pop music without pretensions, I and several others found this song cloying and banal, and not suited as a tribute to a young man who found mawkishness distasteful, but it did have a certain melodic insistence that could catch one's throat and make one feel the tears prick, especially in circumstances such as these.

The chapel was too small for the two hundred or so who were there. The pews and the aisles were full and there were still people standing outside. The immediate family and closest friends sat in side pews facing the coffin, where their grief could be observed by the rest of the congregation. Such a public position did not make them hold back. 'I can hardly remember a thing that was said I was crying so much,' said Elaine. 'I had to listen to the whole thing on a tape afterwards.' Lee, too, could not let propriety get in the way of his feelings. He was massively and visibly distressed – and, as he recalled to me, he thought he was not going to be: 'I felt really good when I went. I got to the church, I was fine. It was a nice day. Everything had gone the way Clive wanted. I didn't think I'd cry. Then it hit me. It really upset me. I couldn't hold it any more. I'd been holding on so long. It didn't bother me what people thought.' Maureen did not cry, however, not because she did not want to, but because Clive had told her that she must not. 'Clive said to her she had to be strong,' said Lee. 'You could see how hard it was for her, but she wouldn't cry, because she had to be strong, one of us had to be strong.'

Peter Wells, the priest whom Clive had asked to conduct his funeral, said at the start of the service that no one should on any account hold back on grief: 'So many people think that crying's the thing you shouldn't do, but it is exactly the thing you should do, because it is a sign of our love and our deep respect.' Accordingly tearful, we sang Clive's favourite hymn, 'God Moves in a Mysterious Way', the title alone of which – and certainly the words of which – seemed to be an exceptional testament to the firmness of Clive's faith in the face of prodigious odds. It is, after all, a hymn which tells us in no uncertain terms to accept the goodness of God's purpose, however unfathomable. In the circumstances of this young man's death, of course, it was saying that there is a reason for everything, even cancer. Clive's belief in this, in spite of the pain and the heartbreak of the most 'purposeless' of illnesses, was awesome and humbling, and the hymn's profundity and relevance were refreshing after the platitudinous exhortations of the pop song that had preceded it.

Funeral perorations are often so exaggerated that it is almost impossible to associate the person being talked about with the person one knew. The two tributes to Clive – one a sermon given by Peter Wells, the other a eulogy delivered by the newsreader Martyn Lewis – were invigorating for their directness and truth. In their words we recognized the Clive we remembered. Peter Wells spoke fittingly of the 'phenomenal purpose' of Clive's brief life, saying in effect that the greatest achievement of that life was the life itself, that Clive's life was his legacy. 'We need people like Clive,' he said, 'who can love in the face of great danger and great despair.' He was an example and an inspiration simply by *being*, because of 'the courage and the hope to go on', despite the knowledge of the imminence and, in the light of his pain, the undoubted comfort of death.

DEATH

We were told that 'One night at the Royal Marsden, waiting for a nurse to turn him ... he heard a voice and felt a figure standing by his bed, and the voice said, "Is there any reason why you cannot come and join me in my Kingdom tonight?" and Clive said, "No, I can't think of any reason why I shouldn't come with you now."' He had also had the courage to acknowledge the moment of readiness for death, and had said to those closest to him, 'When I am gone, don't worry, for after I have died I will be complete in the Kingdom of God,' and Peter Wells said of this: 'I'm not sure I could say that. I'm not sure that there are many people who could say that, especially when they've suffered so much.'

He asked us to be thankful for the effect of Clive's life upon our lives, and it was this inspiration – the impact of one life upon countless other lives – that Martyn Lewis emphasized too in his eulogy: 'What Clive did in his approach to life was so much more than a personal achievement against overwhelming odds, it was an inspiration to everyone whose lives he touched; whether he was just having a casual conversation, or talking to millions during his appearances on *Breakfast Time* or on *Wogan*, he offered hope and strength to the one in every three people who are going to be told at some time in their lives that they have cancer. He leaves them and all of us a legacy, a shining example of how to live life to the full.' Peter Wells spoke of 'the responsibility to leave this chapel today and to go out with that courage that Clive had, to go out and display that courage and that faith to other people'.

Martyn Lewis also read a poem by Clive called *A Final Goodbye*. It bears little literary distinction, but it could not fail to move because of its relevance to the young man's life and death:

> Why do we search for an answer to what is after death?
> It is fear.
> Fear of the unknown,
> A way of self-preparation in something we shall have no control
>   or say.
> But we never seek to answer what was before birth.

Clive knew that he had come from somewhere and therefore that he was going somewhere. That was his comfort.

The coffin was again raised by the pall-bearers – who included Lee, and Gareth Pyne-James, the founder of Search 88 – and carried out of the chapel. Watching the tear-streaked faces of Clive's immediate family and friends, acknowledging their enormous grief with our own tears, it was impossible not to feel inspired nonetheless, even hopeful, as we all followed the coffin out into the sun after the singing of the twenty-third psalm. Lifted back into the hearse, the coffin was driven slowly through the extensive cemetery towards the waiting open grave, about half a mile from the chapel. The chief mourners followed in another car. We, the rest, ambled slowly and pensively towards the graveside, holding back until the committal had finished in the presence of family and close friends. When all was completed and the coffin had been lowered into the ground, everyone shuffled forward, singly or in small groups, to stand in respect for a few seconds by the grave, looking down at the coffin, conveying mute farewells, and understanding fully as never before perhaps that Clive was inside that box because he was dead and we would never see him again. For many of us, turning away from the grave and, because we were wondering what to do next, looking again at the wreaths now laid along the path by the grave, it was the first time we had seen the wreath from the Duchess of York: 'To a Very Courageous Man. May You Now Rest in Peace. Sarah.'

To me, the most moving aspect of Clive's funeral was the effect it had upon the young people present – those of around Clive's own age, many of whom had never been to a funeral before, or at least not to the funeral of someone to whom they felt so close: his carers, some of whom had travelled hundreds of miles to be there, some of the young actors and actresses who had been in his play, his brother Lee, of course, and Elaine. Compared to their open, stunned, white-faced grief, the mourning of the older generation seemed positively phlegmatic. At the gathering after the funeral at Clive's flat, at which a good deal of alcohol was consumed, and there was laughter, as Clive would have wished, it was the young ones who laughed least, who found it hard even to smile. They had been struck by intimations of mortality as never before, and the loss of one of their own.

Lee said: 'I felt lost. I felt something really big had gone. It was a really big gap.' He had thought that it would be a relief when Clive died, after all the waiting and the anxiety, but when the end came, it was no relief at all: 'It had been hard work, it had stopped all our lives, and sometimes – it sounds nasty but sometimes you think, "Christ, how much longer is this going to go on?" It used to really get me down and you think that even though it'll be sad it'll be a relief, but when it happened it wasn't. It wasn't at all. Everything felt empty.'

When everyone but those closest to the immediate family had left, Maureen broke down. 'She was really bad,' Lee remembered. 'She'd been holding it back for so long.' There were suggestions that she should take some of Clive's Valium, but she refused it. The months of gnawing anxiety, during which she had with such dignity tried to remain cool and controlled, suddenly got the better of her – but what hit her most, just as it hit Lee, was the emptiness, made the worse by the fact that the boy she had just lost was a boy she had only recently got to know. It had been the last six months of Clive's life that had brought him and his mother together, and during that time they had become friends as well as mother and son and they had learnt love for each other.

It was always the recollections of Clive's last days that brought tears to Maureen's eyes, for the simple reason that they were days full of the love of a son for his mother and of a mother for her son. It was for this reason that she could say that she had in a strange sense 'enjoyed' the time, for all the pain: 'I was quite enjoying what I was doing, knowing that I hadn't got to do anything else. I'd told them at work I wasn't coming in any more because I knew Clive hadn't got long to go. Normally when Clive was ill I'd have to be up at the hospital or go and see him at home, twice a week if he wasn't bad, and more if he wasn't well, and I was trying to keep a job going and I used to get so tired and so worn out. So when I gave up work I had all the time in the world to do what I had to do. I didn't have to consider anything else – I didn't even consider Lee really. I never found it hard. There were days when I was tired, but then I used to catch up and get a few hours' kip in the afternoon, and I felt OK. But I think what made it so nice as well was that Clive was so happy, to be at home, and he was so happy to have me looking after him. Because people used to come and if they said, "Oh you look a lot better today, Clive," he'd say, "I know, it's because Mo's looking after me and it's all her good cooking." I remember we washed him down one day, me and Fiona, and he wasn't at all well, and we washed him from head to toe, and we changed all the sheets and we piled all the pillows up and propped him up and brushed his hair, we even shaved him, and he sat down and he looked at me and he said, big smile on his face, "Oh that feels lovely, thanks, Mo."' (Maureen is known to all her close friends as Mo, as she was to Clive.)

In the weeks following Clive's death I found myself talking to those who had been close to him as if he was still alive, using the present tense when referring to him, and they responded in like manner. It did not seem to matter. I never had to pull myself up about it, or apologize. There was also a wonderful openness in all the conversations about him – nothing was glossed over or simply not referred to out of respect for the dead. To be entirely truthful was the ultimate respect. There was a great deal of laughter, as well as quite a few tears, in the remembering. There was nothing hushed and awestruck. Lee noticed this, too, when *he* spoke of his dead brother, not only to me, but to others who were close to Clive: 'We can talk about him and laugh about him without thinking, "Oh, shall I mention him?" With Mum you don't think, "Will it upset her if I talk about him?" She *wants* you to talk about him.'

Lee also noticed that whenever he talked of Clive it was as if he was still alive, as if his brother was not really dead. But the truth hit him one day in the simplest way. Someone he did not know very well, a friend of a friend, was in the flat that Lee and Maureen lived in and noticed a framed photograph of Clive on a shelf: 'And he said, "Who's that?" and I said, "That's my brother," and he said, "Where is he now?" and I said – I didn't like the way I said it. I said it off the top of my head. I said it cold – I said, "He's dead." And you could see it was nothing to him, not really. And that's when it hit. That he *was* dead.'

When Clive died people were not slow to tell Elaine, who had first met him when she was fourteen and he was twelve, and who was now twenty-four years old, that she could 'have her own life now he's gone'. There can be no doubt that she will, but for the moment she must mourn him and miss him. 'I do miss him,' she said to me so often. Beneath an ever-cheerful surface, she knows very acutely that he has gone. She would recall to me how he 'used to call me his sweetheart, his Miss World, when he was in a good mood'. When he was feeling ill-at-ease and frustrated and angry at his circumstances, Elaine would so often be the one he would shout at. She would give him as good as he gave, shouting back at him and walking out in a huff. For forgiveness he would send her roses. 'You've got me round your little finger, I'd say.' More than anyone, I think, she got the sharp end of Clive's sadness, but she accepted it, knowing its significance. 'People told me not to get involved because I'd be so unhappy,' she said, 'but it was such a pleasure, and a privilege'.

2

SICKNESS

CLIVE was killed by an astrocytoma, a tumour of the nervous system, one of the many different tumours that come under the generic term 'glioma', which are tumours that arise in the substance of the brain or in the spinal cord. About half of the tumours of the nervous system are gliomas, and about a quarter of all gliomas are astrocytomas. Only about 2 per cent of deaths from cancer are caused by tumours of the nervous system, and it is far rarer for a tumour to grow in the spinal cord than in the brain. Clive's astrocytoma was lodged in his spinal cord, so his particular tumour was a fairly uncommon one. Clive was aware of this, and would speak of his astrocytoma as being something rather special. 'When they first told me that that was what I'd got, I used to be quite proud of it,' he said. 'I used to say quite proudly, "I've got an astrocytoma."'

The astrocytoma is slow-growing and it is not uncommon in children. It carries a mean survival of about eight years, although Clive survived considerably longer. If the astrocytoma starts to grow inside the spinal cord as opposed to in the brain, then the pressure on the cord itself will eventually cause paralysis, as was the case with Clive. Like almost all gliomas, the astrocytoma is not 'malignant' in the truly technical sense because it does not lead to what are known in medical parlance as metastases, or 'secondaries', in other words the spread of the cancerous process – the uncontrolled division of malignant cells – to other parts of the body. It sits very much on its own, but although *technically* benign, its invidiousness lies in the fact that it is lodged in the brain, or, as with Clive, very close to it, and therefore its growth is bound to cause serious disturbance to the body's activity, and in the last resort it is going to prevent the body functioning at all. This is what happened to Clive. His astrocytoma, on the night of Tuesday 1 March, finally did what it had threatened to do for many years – having extended upward beyond the spinal cord into the brain stem, it invaded that part of the stem known as the medulla, or more specifically the medulla oblongata, which contains the centres in the brain which control certain vital bodily processes like respiration and cardiovascular activity, and so it was that Clive blacked out and his heart stopped.

His tumour was particularly nasty, too, in that the pain it caused, being pain resulting from nerve damage, was never fully controllable. Neuralgic pain is always unpredictable and there is no knowing how it will react, if at all, to the administration of various drugs. One of the finest cancer hospitals in the world, the Royal Marsden Hospital, with all its expertise in pain control and its carefully controlled dispensation of extremely powerful drugs, was unable fully to remove Clive's agony, which was intense, and, to the mind of the comparatively healthy, unimaginable. Like all neuralgic cancer patients, a level of pain was something that Clive had to learn to live with. It is sadly not true that cancer pain is always avoidable with the right treatment – although an inclination to misinterpret the message of the admirable hospice movement has led some to hold this view. Not all cancer patients can live out their last days in an entirely painless state – most can, perhaps, but Clive was not one of them, and it seems that patients who have the extreme misfortune to be the victims of neuralgic tumours cannot be guaranteed freedom from the particularly invasive and excruciating pain that nerve pain is.

The fact that Clive's astrocytoma was lodged in his spinal cord rendered it especially cruel in two other respects: the first, obviously, was that the pressure on the cord meant that paralysis was inevitable; the second was that it was an easily hidden tumour, not at all immediately apparent. Clive never fully understood this, neither did those close to him, and as a result there was resentment that the tumour was not discovered before it was; but it is a sad fact that it was a tumour that was extremely difficult to detect, even under X-ray. This was certainly the case when Clive first began to experience the pain that the tumour caused, which was some eight years before it was found; and even when it was found it could not be diagnosed with certainty because scanning equipment was simply not sophisticated enough, to begin with to see it at all, and latterly to identify it positively. In fact a CT-scan performed on Clive comparatively recently was still not capable of displaying the full extent of the tumour, so embedded was it, and advances in the nature of scanning in the fifteen years since Clive's astrocytoma first made itself felt have been substantial.

At the age of seven, Clive had a slight accident which he remembered vividly as the start of all his troubles, although it is by no means certain that it was actually the cause of anything in itself. He was walking home from school one day when for a reason he could not recall he briefly stepped off the pavement into the road and was hit by a passing car. He was struck from behind, but not hard enough to cause any obvious damage, as the car was moving very slowly. He did fall to the ground, however. The driver of the car got out to see if he was all right. Clive got up, brushed himself down, and continued on his way home. There was apparently no immediate pain, but he was quite shocked, and when he reached home he hid for a while in the garden shed. Returning from shopping, his mother heard of the accident from a neighbour. She was not unduly alarmed as nothing was broken and Clive did not seem to be in any pain – she remembered that he was playing on the swing in the back garden when she arrived home. The matter was soon forgotten.

A couple of months after the accident, Clive started to wake up in the middle of the night screaming. He was experiencing excruciating pain – 'a kind of insistent throbbing' – in the back of his neck. The local doctor was summoned several times, but it was unfortunate and seemed unfair that each time he arrived the pain had abated. Unable to diagnose anything, he gave Clive aspirin, and subsequently stronger painkillers like Distalgesic, but nothing helped when the pain was at its worst. One night the pain was so extreme, and Clive's screaming so loud and prolonged, that he was taken to the casualty department of his local hospital where he was X-rayed – the first of the innumerable X-rays in his short life. Nothing was found, either on this or several ensuing visits. He was then examined more thoroughly in the orthopaedic department of another hospital, where further X-rays were taken, and still nothing was found – and it was recommended that he commence psychiatric treatment. 'They couldn't explain it so they put it down to emotional upset,' said Clive. The symptoms were ascribed to the trauma that it was assumed he was undergoing as a result of the chaotic and sad state of his parents' marriage, which had been rocky almost from the moment it began, and which, with a timing that seemed significant, had broken down irretrievably shortly after Clive had had his little accident. He and his mother, and his younger brother, had had to move into a 'prefab' in Peckham in South London, where they lived with his maternal grandmother.

For a while Clive diligently visited a psychiatrist once a week. He could not remember anything about these visits except that there seemed to be 'a lot of playing with toys'. The pain did not go away. The severe attacks, which sometimes did not restrict themselves to the neck area but radiated down his back, would occur for about a week every eight weeks, usually at night or upon waking in the morning; but a chronic, rumbling, dull pain was there all the time. Talking to Clive about this pain, I asked him if he had experienced worse pain since, and he replied that he undoubtedly had, indeed that it had been very much worse, but that there was a difference: 'Now, at least, however bad it is, at least it's believed and it's explainable, which makes it better somehow, although it's really worse. In the early days no one seemed to believe me, so they wouldn't give me anything, except something like Distalgesic which just didn't touch it. It was always as if I was making a fuss about nothing very serious.'

Clive must have felt very alone with his pain, apparently unbelieved and unsupported – except by his parents, it has to be said, both of whom had a fundamental layperson's disrespect for psychologists and psychology – 'My father particularly had no time for them, from the word go really. He was old-fashioned and he just didn't trust them.' Clive's mother was more baffled than aggressively sceptical, not quite grasping that an extreme pain, however real it may be to its victim, can still be psychosomatic in origin: 'It was there, you could see it, he was screaming, he wasn't making it up,' she said. 'How could they say it wasn't real?'

Presumably no psychiatrist was saying that the pain was not genuine, only that its origins may have been in the mind. Clive could never quite grasp this point either – but then he *was* the victim, and he would have had to be superhumanly objective to understand what could well have been a sincere concern on the part of his doctors and psychiatrists to understand the cause of his pain. Neither could he be expected to forgive them for being wrong, as everyone now knows they were, however acceptable their judgement may have been at the time. For there can be no doubt now that what was causing the pain was his astrocytoma, a very physical entity.

The psychosomatic solution was so avidly pursued at this time, however, that Clive was admitted to a children's psychiatric unit at another hospital in South East London. In recalling the place to me, Clive described a kind of juvenile Bedlam, a peculiar sort of children's hell: 'The kids were loony, uncontrollable, and most of them were on drugs or sedated. The ward, so that they could make more room for play facilities during the day, had beds that went up into the walls, and there was a boy next to me who was totally mad. My grandmother used to visit me at this place and she'd always bring chocolates and sweets, and this boy used to get all my sweets because he used to say to me, "If you don't give me all your sweets I'll push your bed up in the middle of the night," and I used to live in fear of being pushed up and squashed like a fly against the wall. I was only eight so the thought was terrifying.' Clive was at this hospital for about a month, 'which seemed so long to a small boy', until his father took him away. The weekly psychiatric visits continued though, as did the pain.

When Clive was ten, three years after the accident and the onset of pain, for most of which time he had been treated psychiatrically, his back was examined, he was again X-rayed, and at last something physically wrong was diagnosed. This was scoliosis, or curvature of the spine. He was fitted with a brace, called a Milwaukee brace, which covered the whole of his back, from the hips right up to the neck, in the hope that the spine would straighten itself as he grew. He wore a series of braces for the next three years. The full term for the malformation of the spine from which Clive suffered was 'idiopathic juvenile scoliosis'. 'Idiopathic' means, simply, that there is no known cause for a particular ailment, and it is a word that is used in the great majority of cases of spinal curvature. In fact, with medical hindsight, it is almost certain that Clive's scoliosis was caused by his astrocytoma. At the time, though, it would have required a huge leap of the medical imagination to make such a remote connection, as the incidence of tumours causing scoliosis is very low, and as nothing could in any case be detected under X-ray. It nonetheless does seem a little strange, and Clive and his family certainly thought it so, that there seemed to be no explanation for the continued pain that Clive was experiencing, since it is also extremely unusual for any kind of pain to be associated with scoliosis. Maureen recalled: 'They kept saying he couldn't be having pain because you don't get pain with scoliosis.'

Clive's pain persisted, although slightly more erratically. Indeed, he could remember periods when he could forget about it altogether, although he had to go on wearing a brace. He was at boarding school now, a preparatory school, which he enjoyed, and he led what he described as a 'very active, independent, boyish life'. But when he was twelve he started to develop a clumsiness in his left leg. 'It kept giving way below my left knee. I'd be walking along and suddenly it'd give way. It was quite frightening. I don't remember any pain when it happened, just shock'. He had to use a walking stick. He was also finding it difficult to urinate, the first sign of the 'bladder problems' which were to become far more serious and highly painful over the years. At this early stage it was merely a case of not being able to 'go' for a while, about ten minutes.

Clive was examined at an orthopaedic hospital in North London. It was concluded that almost three years of wearing braces had had little positive effect. His pain, which was now radiating to his right shoulder and down the length of his spine, was also noted. A major operation was advised. The urinary problems were ascribed to phimosis, the medical term for an overtight foreskin, and circumcision was recommended, although this would have to wait until after the operation. Clive was thoroughly examined for urological infections and everything was reported as normal. It is a fact that a tumour embedded in the spinal cord will often cause urological difficulties, but there was of course no talk of a tumour at this time.

Clive was now thirteen. The operation he had to undergo involved the insertion of a metal rod in his back, called a Harrington rod. The process was called spinal fusion. It was hoped that after the insertion of the rod the spine would quite literally 'fuse' with it, thereby forcing the spine to straighten itself. In preparation for the fusion Clive had to spend time in traction, during which the spine was stretched to the point where it was straight enough for the fusion to be performed. The operation itself was long and complex, involving as it did not only the insertion of the rod, but the removal of bone chips from Clive's hip which were used as part of the fusing process. Clive recalled pain upon coming round from his anaesthetic, but the more distressing memory was of not being allowed to move, of having to lie on his back, and of learning to eat and drink in that prone position. It was his first taste of extreme incapacity. He had to wear a jacket made of plaster, covering his entire upper torso. He was supine, although allowed to push himself around the ward on a trolley, for a month.

About a fortnight after the operation he remembered an attack of severe pain, for which he was X-rayed; he was subsequently told that the fusion had been successful and the rod was secure, although, as he said, 'It wasn't the rod I wanted to know about, it was the pain.' He was discharged from hospital. After the removal of his plaster, he had to wear another Milwaukee brace for about six months, during which time he was circumcised in the hope of solving his urological problems.

Not long after the removal of his brace, and a pronouncement on the part of those who had performed the fusion that it was 'perfect', Clive tripped over a step at his school and experienced pain in the lumbar region, or lower part of the spine. He was admitted to hospital with a fever and continual pain and difficulty of movement in his left hip. He had a biopsy in the area of his groin, which was reported as normal. He was sent to another hospital for a bone scan. According to Clive, one of the doctors involved noticed a 'hot spot' on the scan at the top of his spine and base of his skull. A 'hot spot' often indicates the presence of a neurological complication of some sort. But Clive thought that the scan seemed to concentrate only on the area around his hip. In this matter one only has his word, and his memory might have been hazy, because there was also talk of a 'hot area' around the hip, and the presence of an 'active bony disease' which might possibly be synovitis, an illness involving the fluid between the joints. Following this prognosis another biopsy was taken in the hip area, but once more the exploration was declared normal. Clive was left with two painful scars as a result of the biopsies. As far as the pain in his hip was concerned, it was recommended that he should commence a course of physiotherapy, which he underwent, and enjoyed, because it involved swimming, an activity he found very pleasant.

Shortly before his fifteenth birthday, almost two years after the insertion of the rod in his back, Clive was readmitted to the orthopaedic hospital at which the fusion had been performed, complaining of sweating at night and a temperature, feeling terribly ill and weak. Although there were to be minor temporary improvements after this, the readmission marked the start of a slow and remorseless deterioration in Clive's health, causing a realization on the part of the doctors that there was something very wrong indeed. On this visit the examining surgeon noticed a wasting of the leg and thighs and a certain amount of pain on movement of these limbs, and it was suggested that these might be the symptoms of incipient paraplegia.

It was decided that Clive should have a myelogram, an X-ray involving the injection of a dye called metrizamide into the space around the spinal cord. Clive told me that it was common to perform myelograms prior to spinal fusions, which meant, in his opinion, that he should have had one two years previously, before the insertion of his rod; in that case, he thought, something might have been discovered then. Unfortunately for Clive's case, it seems not to be routine for myelography to be carried out prior to such operations, especially if there are no obvious symptoms of neurological disturbance at the time, and the doctors concluded that there were none. Besides which, even if a myelogram *had* been performed then, it is debatable that anything would have been found.

As it was, nothing was found on *this* myelogram, even now, when doctors were discovering for the first time real and potentially disturbing neurological symptoms. The reason that nothing was found – if Clive's recollections and his medical notes covering this period are to be believed – was that for some still unexplained reason the results of this myelogram seemed to concentrate only on the middle and lower, or the lower thoracic and lumbar, regions of the spine, and not upon the area around the astrocytoma, which was in the upper part of the spine, or the lower thorax.

After this, Clive was advised to resume his psychiatric treatment. He recalled to me that his father nearly exploded at the suggestion, but eventually succumbed, and Clive began to see a psychologist attached to the hospital. For a short while, in his sadness and desperation, he started to be tempted to believe that the psychosomatic solution might be correct: 'Part of me wanted to believe that they were right, especially when so many people, after all that time, had been telling me there was nothing there. But at the same time I knew I had pain, and that one day they'd find out what was really causing it.'

A couple of months after being discharged from hospital, Clive had to be readmitted because of a suspected complication around the upper part of his rod. He had felt a click as he was getting out of the bath, and the onset of severe pain. He was X-rayed and told yet again that the rod was secure and in position, that it had not shifted in any way, as had been suspected. What he was not told – at least he did not recall being told – was that the X-ray had at least covered the part of the upper thorax that the results of the myelogram appeared to have failed to cover, and that there was indeed an enlargement of the spinal canal of some sort in that area.

No immediate action seemed to be taken as a result. Perhaps this did not matter in the overall scheme of things, because it was only a few months before something more definite *was* found and noted, and action was taken, although in the interim Clive had to endure, without even the briefest respite it seems, an enormous decline in his general health. It started with a frightening deterioration in the urological area. He had continued to have difficulty in urinating ever since the circumcision, but had always managed it eventually, with patience and discomfort. Now he suddenly could not urinate at all. 'I'd just been to see the film of *Macbeth* with the school. I'd been wanting to go all evening, but we weren't allowed to go during the film and then after the film when I had a chance to go I just couldn't, and it went on until it became unbearable. So we went to the casualty department of the nearest hospital, and they told me I'd need a catheter. I didn't know what on earth they meant.' Clive had to experience yet another kind of agony, the pain of catheterization. This was to be the first of many – some thirty in all, he thought – that he would have to undergo in the ensuing years. 'Actually the worst pain isn't when they put it in, it's when they pull it out.' He was also subjected to several urological tests after this first catheterization, which he described as 'painful and traumatic'.

Clive then suffered a Christmas which he told me was the worst he could remember. He was bedbound for most of it, and on Christmas Day he was attacked by the severest neck and back pain he had ever felt. The deep agony would keep him awake at night and he was given pethidine, which helped him to sleep somewhat but did not really take away the pain. He was continuing to have problems emptying his bladder, so that was causing him pain too. He was losing weight, soaking his bedclothes at night with sweat, and vomiting. When he stood up, he kept falling down. He was of course permanently and massively tired.

He was admitted yet again to the orthopaedic hospital where he had had the fusion and where he was now examined by a neurologist he had not met before, who, after performing various tests, concluded – though not as yet to Clive or to his relatives – that he unquestionably had a 'lesion' in the upper thoracic region of the spine. 'Lesion' is of course a term with a very wide application, covering as it can any impairment of tissue from the smallest cut to the most savage tumour. The neurologist, expressing some surprise to his colleagues, though not to Clive, that the previous myelogram had not seemed to cover the relevant area of the spine, recommended that a second myelogram be undertaken – which it was, without delay, and this time the results covered the entire spine, including the upper thoracic and cervical regions. Sure enough, a very extensive lesion was discovered in Clive's spinal cord, stretching from the cervix to the lower thorax.

At this stage it was impossible to give a precise name to the newly discovered growth. Clive found out later that theories abounded as to what it might be, and the possibility of its being a tumour, or specifically a 'slow-growing glioma', was not discounted. It was not possible to subject the growth to further radiological examination immediately, because the dye left in from the myelogram would have interfered with any image. Whatever the theories and the terms being passed to and fro between the experts out of Clive's hearing, Clive remembered being told that he had a 'cyst' which would have to have an eye kept on it, but that his fusion was 'fine'.

Clive burst into tears. They were not tears of fear or panic or sorrow, only of exhaustion and relief. The indeterminate and unthreatening word 'cyst' seemed solid and reassuring, because what mattered was 'to be believed at last, and to be told that there was something there'. This 'cyst', as far as Clive could comprehend, had been the cause of eight years of pain. He had also prayed the night before the myelogram, and his prayer seemed to have been answered. He had always been a religious boy, but this was the first time he had offered up such a blunt prayer with regard to his illness: 'Lord, you know I am not imagining the pain and that there is something wrong, so please help the doctors find out what it is.'

Clive's father was far from satisfied. He was especially angered by the idea that, as far as he could tell, all that was going to happen next was that Clive's 'cyst' was going to have an eye kept on it. He felt that he and his son did not have the time for the deliberations between doctors that such an important diagnosis unavoidably entailed. Clive recalled that his father caused quite a dramatic scene, berating the entire medical profession, including of course the psychiatrists, as liars and charlatans. He then said he was discharging his son from the hospital and that they were going to get a second opinion.

Clive's local doctor recommended that he be seen separately by two distinguished neurosurgeons. Both surgeons agreed as to the presence of a lesion, and both, significantly, said that judging from its size it must have been there for some considerable time. It was at this stage too that Clive discovered that the lesion, whatever it was specifically, was almost certainly what had caused his supposedly 'idiopathic' scoliosis. Where the two surgeons disagreed was on the matter of how urgent it was that something be done to remove, or attempt to remove, the growth. For the first time there was talk of a threat to Clive's life. One surgeon recommended an operation as soon as possible or, as Clive remembered being told, 'I couldn't be expected to live much longer. I was given about a year.' Surprisingly, he did not remember being unduly startled by this prognosis: 'Perhaps I didn't really take it in. All I remember thinking was that they were going to give me another operation, and I'd had so many operations that one more didn't seem to make much difference, except that this one, I thought, was going to take away the pain.' He claimed that he was in fact so assured by the surgeon, in so many words: 'He told me he was going to cure the pain.' Clive also recalled asking about the risks involved. He was told, he said, that there were inevitable risks in all operations and was warned that he might experience a slight paralysis, but that this would only be temporary.

He was admitted for surgery to the neurological hospital to which the neurosurgeon who had expressed urgency was attached. Movingly, he recalled to me the night before his operation: 'They always say before an operation that they want you to empty your bowels, that they want you to "go". Well I just couldn't. The only way I knew of "going" was just to walk around, and for some reason that night I just couldn't stop walking around. I walked around from the time my grandmother and my dad left at the end of visiting hours, about nine or half past nine, until the next morning almost. I just couldn't sleep. I just walked around. I had coffee with the night staff downstairs in the canteen, I walked around the whole hospital. It was a dingy place, not a modern hospital at all. It was a very old building, very antiquated, with tiny wards. It was like a Victorian workhouse really. And I walked around the whole place, and all around the outside. I literally walked around all night, just walking.'

When Clive came round from the operation the next day he found himself in the hospital's intensive care unit and in extreme pain. He had to be turned occasionally, which was even more painful. He noticed that his hair had been 'chopped about', which annoyed him because he had just had what he considered to be rather a good haircut. And he could not seem to move his legs, or feel one leg on top of the other. Because he could not sit up or move his neck, he could not check to see if he actually had any legs. He had to ask someone if his legs were still there. He was told he was suffering from paraplegia, but that it was only temporary. With physiotherapy the feeling in his legs would come back. He was also informed that upon examination of his lesion under anaesthetic it had been decided that it would not be wise even to attempt to remove it because of the risk to the surrounding nerves. All that it had been possible to do was to perform a biopsy. The growth would have to be subjected to a course of radiotherapy.

Radiotherapy involves the bombardment of the tumour with radiation in order to shrink it or at least to retard its growth. For his treatment Clive was admitted to the Royal Marsden Hospital in the Fulham Road. No one had yet mentioned the word 'cancer' in his presence, neither did he remember thinking at the time that he might actually have cancer, even though he knew well enough that the hospital he was entering was most particularly a cancer hospital. It was indeed the country's leading and most celebrated one, especially at the time Clive was admitted, when it was very much in the news because of its association with the jockey Bob Champion and his 'fight for life'. Clive could not recall any fear or concern upon arriving at the Marsden, but rather a kind of pride, and a sense of privilege. It was not long either before he recognized that he was in a caring and trustworthy environment, and an unusually open one too, which must have been a relief to him: 'You got the feeling that you could ask questions and they'd be answered.' He also discovered that the Marsden was a very Christian hospital, and because of the strength of his own belief he found that a special comfort. He had not been there long before he was christened and confirmed on the same day, Good Friday.

His happy memories of this time – bonding friendships with members of staff that were to last the rest of his life, a general feeling of being in considerate, expert hands – may of course have had something to do with the conviction he still held that his tumour, for it was now spoken of as a tumour, would go away and he would walk again; he always talked of the Marsden as an impressively 'good' place, though, even recalling his many subsequent visits, when he knew there was no hope of a cure. It was nonetheless touching that he could remember the Marsden with such affection when it was there that he first had to undergo the traumatic experience of radiotherapy, and later chemotherapy.

He was subjected to radiotherapy every day for three months. Even though this was the first clinical experience he had undergone that did not seem to involve any pain, he recalled it as being peculiarly grim and frightening. Because it was extremely painful for Clive to lie on his stomach, the tumour could not be attacked directly from behind. Rather the beam had to be directed through his neck with crucial exactitude to the precise spot, and for this he had to have a plastic mask made, for which he initially had to have a cast. Then he had to be secured to the machine with the mask on his face – 'and they left me alone, because it was dangerous, in this room with walls six feet thick to stop the radiation'. He heard a faint humming and felt a slight burning sensation in his throat. 'I was terribly frightened.'

As Clive began to get used to the fearful claustrophobia of the treatment, the side-effects started to make themselves felt – a difficulty in swallowing, extreme nausea, loss of hair, and a general overwhelming weakness, which worsened as the months passed. His pain had lessened, but he had never felt so monstrously ill before. What kept him going, he recollected, was his faith and a sustained consumption of sedatives and painkillers – some of them illicit, in that he used to save his night-time sleeping pills to take during the day at the moments when the sickness became too bad.

It was at the Marsden that Clive's tumour was diagnosed as an astrocytoma. No hope can have been held out for a cure, and the radiotherapy served a solely palliative function; the best that could be expected was a slowing-down of the tumour's growth. Clive did not remember being given this unfavourable outlook, but then neither could he remember asking about it at the time. He existed, understandably, on optimism. As far as he was concerned his tumour was being cured. Why else the wretchedness of radiotherapy? His assumption that this was the case can only have been strengthened when he found himself discharged from the Marsden and readmitted to the hospital at which his operation had been performed, where there was no further talk of tumours or of any form of treatment now except physiotherapy. 'Their aim,' said Clive, 'was to get me fit at any cost,' and, he presumed, walking again.

Because of the radiotherapy, the after-effects of which lasted for months, he was still feeling appallingly weak and sick, but he battled on with what was required of him – a series of hard and exhausting physical exercises which must have seemed excessively gruelling for someone so very tired and ill. The three months at the Marsden had also weakened his limbs, since between the bouts of treatment he had done nothing much more than lie down and sleep. Also he was no longer on effective painkillers, so the hard physical activity increased his pain.

So began an intensively painful and confusing year – 'the *worst* year of my life', Clive remembered. The confusion was caused by what seemed to him to be conflicting opinions as to the state of his paralysis. Having been told that it would only be temporary, the impression was now being given by some physiotherapists that there was very little chance that he would ever walk again. The first time he was given this opinion he was so shattered by it that he had to be put on Valium.

The physiotherapy continued and he did not know what to believe, especially when he started to experience some slight physical improvement – 'I'd been through hell, being dragged to physiotherapy even when I was feeling absolutely appalling, I'd had all kinds of infections, my bladder still wasn't working properly, giving me a lot of pain, my neck pain was going on, but because I was starting to be able to move things a bit more easily than I could before, I really did think I was on the mend, that everything was going to be all right, that the tumour was going away, that it had probably gone, and that I'd be walking.' Possibly he believed all this, as is so often the case, because he wanted to believe it. At one point towards the end of this year of physiotherapy someone suggested to Clive that he go to Stoke Mandeville Hospital for more rigorous and specialized treatment. 'That shocked me, because I didn't think the situation was bad enough to warrant it. Stoke Mandeville's the place where the really bad cases go. I didn't think I was that bad a case.'

One cause of pain during this time had an air of farce about it, in spite of the agony involved. Clive certainly talked of it with some amusement. He was experiencing kyphosis, which is a convexity in the curvature of the spine, observable to the naked eye when the torso is looked at from the side. He was also experiencing neck pain that was more intense than usual, and it was noticed that the lump at the back of his neck at the top of the spine seemed to be increasing in size daily. It was, in fact, and quite alarmingly simply, the top of the Harrington rod which was beginning to penetrate the skin and poke through the back of Clive's neck. He had to have the top of the rod 'cut off' – 'if they'd let it go on any longer, you'd have seen the rod sticking out!'

Out of the confusion of this period there arose a desperate act that was also recollected with some relish, combining as it did the comic with the thrill of a certain amount of danger. Its implications, however, were far from amusing. Concluding that there was only one way of finding out the truth, and that that was to have a proper look at Clive's medical notes, Clive, his mother and grandmother decided to steal them. A first attempt to steal the notes was unsuccessful because Clive's grandmother's courage failed at the last minute, but a second effort was fruitful, and the notes were filched, taken to an off-licence close to the hospital, copied on a photocopier there, and returned to their rightful place in the office all during the course of one suppertime. 'We had so many bits of paper,' Clive's mother recalled, 'that the man in the off-licence kept looking at us suspiciously, so I had to tell him that we were two secretaries from the hospital and that the hospital copier had broken down.'

The notes revealed much that Clive had not known before, a

55

lot of which has already been dealt with in the telling of this sad story. Most significantly, in his view, he learnt for the first time about the differences in opinion as to the nature of his tumour, perhaps inevitable at the time that they were recorded, and some concern on the part of certain contributors to the notes that it had not been discovered sooner than it was. Whatever the truth of this diagnosis, or the complexities of opinion involved, it was disturbing indeed for Clive to read, as he did now, that this thing that was causing him to be confined to a wheelchair, to which some people were saying he would be restricted for life, might possibly have been found earlier than it in fact had been. And if it had been discovered sooner, he had to ask himself, would there have been a better chance of its successful removal? 'For the first time,' Clive said, 'the word "negligence" started to whirl around in my head.'

Clive kept his discoveries and thoughts to himself for the moment – 'I just wasn't brave enough to tell anyone we'd nicked the notes' – and he continued with his physiotherapy. After a purgatorial year of this, under intolerable circumstances, he was told, unanimously and crushingly, that there was no point in continuing the treatment because there was definitely no improvement in his physical condition, and that he might as well resign himself to remaining in a wheelchair for ever. Clive needed confirmation from a source other than 'a bunch of physios and occupational therapists that I hardly knew', and he went to see the neurosurgeon who had performed the biopsy.

Clive had matured considerably in the past two years or so – he was seventeen and old enough to demand truthful answers, if too young still to realize that medicine is as full of uncertainties as anything else. So for his persistence he was reluctantly given a very frightening prognosis. Apparently he was told that the improvements that had been hoped for had clearly not occurred and that he was indeed going to be confined to a wheelchair from now on; and, according to Clive, the tumour was mentioned again for the first time in a long time, with alarming connotations: 'He gave me four years. He said it just like that. "The best you can hope for in the next four years is that you'll stay as you are, in the wheelchair, or that you'll die."'

I have to emphasize at this stage in this bleak narrative that it was only Clive who recollected these precise words; his mother, who Clive told me was with him when the prognosis was made, cannot remember them. She recalls that the surgeon held out little hope for recovery, but not that he gave any kind of exact timespan for Clive's future – and it was hardly something, if it had been so definite, that she would be likely to forget. Also, after this 'final diagnosis' as Clive liked to call it, he himself did not immediately accept the full import of what had been said; as far as his disability was concerned, at least, the next move on his part seemed to be to prove wrong those physiotherapists who had told him that there was no point in continuing with the efforts to improve his physical condition. He subjected himself to another year of physiotherapy, first as an outpatient at his local hospital, where he did not seem to experience much improvement; he was eventually told by a doctor there that he was 'plateauing out', and that what he should do with the time that was left to him was to stop the physiotherapy and 'get himself a decent education at a good university'. Clive's response to this advice was instant resistance: 'I thought that if I had a limited time I wanted to achieve as much as possible in that time, and I didn't want to waste it behind some desk. I needed to grow up as quickly as possible.'

It was while he was undergoing physiotherapy as an outpatient that he saw a television programme about an organization called the National Association for Compensation Claimants. He wrote to the founder of the Association, Pat Carter. His letter began: 'I am seventeen years old and suffering, both physically and psychologically, as a result of what I believe is incompetence and neglect of the way I was treated, medically.' Clive's bitterness at this time led him to give the impression in the letter that he was accusing *all* those who had treated him of neglect, although of course many of the doctors and nurses with whom he had come into contact had devoted great care and attention to him.

He described, in eight pages of careful and painful detail, his medical history from the time of his accident at the age of seven. He quoted at length from the notes he had purloined. He was clearly somewhat confused as to where precisely he wanted to claim medical negligence. His sense of suffering and overall distress at his situation was so acute that he just wanted to put it all down, the whole terrible story. 'I didn't want to blame anyone really. I wasn't interested in blame. I just wanted to know why I'd ended up the way I had. It seemed unfair.' The letter ended with a heartbreaking description of his overall state:

I have numerous problems, severe pain, discomfort and am VERY dependent on help, even to do the simplest task. My problems include:

1. Severe neck pain – restricting sitting to about two hours.
2. Ever present soreness over possible pressure areas.
3. Impaired bladder function.
4. No bowel motion – needing three enemas a week and manual evacuation.
5. Breathing problems.
6. Risk to infections, especially urinary, and viruses.

I am now partially tetraplegic, weakness over all the body. The quality of my life has diminished beyond all recognition. Instead of seventeen being the age of independence and exploring life, education, jobs etc., it is the complete reverse.

Clive's letter provoked an immediate response, and he was contacted by a firm of solicitors willing to act for him in any claim for negligence. They said he had a strong case in that there seemed to be an argument that the tumour could have been, indeed should have been, found earlier than it was, and that if it had been operated upon at that early stage the deterioration he had experienced since might not have been inevitable. The inquiries continued for over a year and, until the last moment, were encouraging in their findings.

Clive continued with his physiotherapy. In spite of all that he had been told, he was obsessed with the possibility of walking again. 'I still couldn't believe what they'd said about me not being able to walk. I was determined to walk, I was engrossed with the idea of walking. I didn't care about improving my mind, and I didn't much care about the lack of movement in my hands and fingers, it was my legs that I was concerned about – all I wanted to do was walk. I thought, "If I can walk again there'll be some point in carrying on."' He asked to be sent to Stoke Mandeville, the hospital he had previously rejected as being a place 'only for the really bad cases'.

Stoke seemed to be very interested in him. He was an unusual case, after all, or as Clive put it, 'not your average spinal cord injury'. He was there for five months, throwing himself with concentrated vigour into physical self-betterment. He remembered a fair amount of substantial pain, which was found to be caused by one vertebra in his spine pressing down on another. He wrote to a friend at this time: 'The doctors want to start messing me around again, carrying out tests and operating on the spine, but I am refusing as I feel I've just been messed around too much already.' Nonetheless he underwent another operation, his last ever, a laminectomy, which relieved the vertebral problem, and there was a marked decrease in the pain.

In fact, after leaving Stoke Mandeville and for about eight months, Clive felt 'almost normal' by his standards (which by any others might be deemed almost unbearable). The physiotherapy had definitely brought about an improvement: 'I was practically standing up. I had to support myself, with one hand on the table, but I was standing.' And the pain, for a while, had abated. There was always a residue of pain in Clive's existence, but in his terms it was barely there any more. As for the tumour, 'I thought it was all in the past, I thought it had gone.'

For a short time, life had the comparative ordinariness and contentment that he had yearned for. This proved to be a highly creative period, and it was now that he started to write a play about a young man in a similar situation to his own, who had cancer and was in a wheelchair. Before he had written a word of it he decided to give it an ironic title – *The Best Years of Your Life*. He was eighteen years old, and living with his grandmother, with whom, because of his family situation, he had been living, when not in hospital or away at school, for ten years. They were about to move out of the 'prefab' into a brand new council flat, with special disabled facilities, a few streets away.

Suddenly things went very wrong indeed, and very rapidly. Clive's grandmother, his 'nan' as he called her, fell ill with a throat infection. Clive was visiting the Royal Marsden at this time – not as a patient but as a researcher for his play. He remembered how the staff at the Marsden had looked at his grandmother with some concern, remarking how thin she looked. She told them about her throat, and it was the Marsden staff who persuaded her that she should go and see her doctor. With reluctance she did, and Clive went with her: 'He said it was the life-change, he told her it was "something women go through", which was odd, since she was over sixty.'

Her condition deteriorated to the point of not being able to swallow anything, and then she began to cough up blood. An X-ray revealed a tumour in the throat. She was first admitted to her local hospital, but knowing of the Marsden's reputation and because of its associations with her loved grandson, she asked to be sent there. She underwent radiotherapy and chemotherapy. Clive had to watch her go through what he had gone through a year and a half before, although he himself had not as yet experienced chemotherapy. That imbalance was soon to be rectified.

Within a few weeks of his grandmother's admission Clive's tumour – forgotten, in effect, for so long – began to make its baleful presence known again, by attacking him with a series of violent and uncontrollable spasms in his chest and one of his shoulders. There was pain too, but Clive was most frightened by the spasms, a symptom he had suffered before, but never as savagely as this. It was a clear indication, of course, of a major interference with the spinal cord, caused by a serious progression in the growth of his tumour. The radiotherapy of eighteen months previously had clearly had a successful palliative effect in that period, but this was obviously now wearing off. The treatment recommended this time was chemotherapy, for which Clive was readmitted to the Marsden – 'So there I was with my nan.'

The aims of chemotherapy and radiotherapy are similar, but the former treatment endeavours to suppress the cancerous process through the administration of potent cell-destroying drugs, by tablet or injection. A treatment that involves the destruction of cells is bound to produce unpleasant side-effects. It has to be

said at this point that many cancer patients undergo chemotherapy with relatively little discomfort, but this is dependent
upon the nature of their cancer. Neuralgic tumours like Clive's
require especially toxic drugs with particularly virulent results.
Clive remembered that the full effects of his first experience of
chemotherapy took a while to work through, and that to begin
with what he had heard seemed to be worse than what he was
feeling. But things did eventually reach such a state of nausea
and overwhelming malaise that he asked for the treatment to be
stopped. 'There's always a point,' he said, 'when the side-effects
seem to outweigh the benefits,' which is the cancer patient's
modest way of saying that the sickness has become so extreme
that it is unendurable, and that the pain caused by the cancer
might be a preferable alternative. Also, while Clive may have
bravely played down the effects of this first course of treatment, it
is significant that when asked if he wanted it again about two
years later, and the alternative he was facing on that occasion
was very probable death, he still had to think very hard as to
which was the more attractive prospect.

In addition to the increasingly debilitating symptoms of his
own treatment, Clive had to watch his grandmother go through
both her radiotherapy and chemotherapy in the same hospital.
She then had to have an operation, in which her voice-box was
removed. 'I remember going to see her in the ironically named
"recovery" room. She was surrounded by machines, pumps and
drips and she couldn't speak any more, and she'd always talked,
she'd always been a great talker, you couldn't get her to stop.
And it was either me who said it to her, or she wrote it down for
me, I can't remember, that she'd been my legs for all those years
and now I was going to have to be her voice.' She died, very soon
and mercifully, after the operation.

Shortly after her death, Clive learnt of the failure of his case for
medical negligence. The proceedings had reached the point of a
writ being drawn up, though not served (as there was considerable uncertainty as to which of the many members of the medical
profession who had treated Clive it should be served upon), but at
the last moment it was concluded that even if there had been
negligence in the tumour not being discovered earlier, the

discovery would have made no difference in any case to Clive's deteriorating condition. In other words, whatever negligence there might have been could not be said to have actively contributed to Clive's ill-health, so he did not have a case in law for a claim. What was in effect being said was that the tumour would not have been wholly removable or curable at whatever stage in Clive's life it had been found, and that his slow decline towards paralysis and death was inescapable from the very beginning.

Bravely, Clive threw himself with fervour into living as full a life as possible within the inevitable limitations. Recalling the rejection of his case he said: 'I didn't know the first thing about law, and neither did anyone else I knew, and I suppose I should have asked more questions, but at the time I was fed up with the whole business and I thought it was more important to get on with things, to get on with life. I was feeling quite well, quite bright.' The most distasteful effects of chemotherapy were wearing off, and its benefits were making themselves apparent. Clive was also experiencing a new freedom, a first taste of adulthood in a way, in that he was living in his own flat. He finished his play. He arranged a trip to the West Coast of America for himself, visiting Hollywood and Disneyland.

Throughout this 'bright' time, which lasted, with the occasional relapse and readmission to the Royal Marsden, for a year and a half, Clive was being helped by drugs to lessen the pain, the most significant of which was diamorphine. Since the time of his radiotherapy, which had been followed by a short regimen of liquid morphine, he had not been on any morphine-based drugs, largely because of an assumption on his part and on the part of the hospitals that he attended other than the Marsden (although Stoke Mandeville offered him diamorphine and he refused it) that he would become addicted, and that they would have a detrimental effect on his mental capacity. 'I wanted my brain to be clear, mainly because of the writing.' It was only when he went into the Marsden for chemotherapy that he was enlightened as to the true effects of morphine when administered to patients in extreme pain. He was told that the pain itself would in a sense absorb the full impact of the drug and that there would, to put it in layman's terms, 'be none left' to have an effect on the rest of the body or its abilities – his cognitive ability would remain un-hampered. In any case, the Royal Marsden was progressive enough to understand that addiction has more to do with the personality of the addict than with the drug itself.

Clive found this piece of illumination a great relief, of course, and he was actually on diamorphine – administered in tablet form – for the rest of his life. It is important and instructive to realize that he was taking diamorphine when he wrote the major part of his play. It did not take away all his pain – his very particular tumour saw to that – but it certainly lessened it, so much so that once on diamorphine he regretted bitterly that he had not been made to understand its true effects much earlier. Another means of relieving his pain was his 'little machine', known as the TENS machine, or the transcutaneous electrical nerve stimulator. This is a device which acts as a counter-irritant by sending tiny electrical impulses into the patient's body through two small electrode pads attached to the back of the neck. Clive himself had control over the amount of impulse he could adminis-ter to himself by adjusting two small dials, and this action would activate the body's own pain-relieving system accordingly.

With the help of his diamorphine – two 10-milligram tablets, then four, and finally six, four times a day – together with various other drugs, and his pain machine, Clive managed to live a com-paratively reasonable life, as far as his health was concerned at any rate. These were undoubtedly his 'best years', sociable, lively, creative. It would be wrong to give the impression that there were no black moments during this period – indeed he could become appallingly depressed, to the point sometimes of con-templating suicide; but his despondency was largely caused by the frustrations of life in a wheelchair and by the personal sadness of his situation – not by any marked deterioration in his health. Once again the tumour did not make its presence felt too severely, or at least not in any noticeably more extreme manner, for a good long while.

But it attacked again, with characteristic suddenness, causing once more an outbreak of furious and unmanageable spasms and a massive increase in the amount of pain. The pain and the spasms were controlled first, then Clive was given a CT-scan and told that there had been a further serious progression of the tumour in that it was starting to invade his brain stem. He was also told, frankly, that little hope could be held out for him if he did not undergo another course of chemotherapy. 'They told me,' said Clive, 'that I might make it until Christmas,' and Christmas was a couple of months away. For the first time in a life of pain and anguish, Clive found himself terrified at the prospect of imminent death. Although he had lived with the possibility of dying too soon ever since 'the final diagnosis', until now he had somehow not been hit by the reality of it. To a certain extent a combination of his youth and his faith had held that reality at bay. He certainly needed his faith now.

'It suddenly seemed real,' said Clive. 'It was the first time I'd been really afraid. Until then I'd thought of death as being a welcome release and an end to all the pain.' Suddenly words like that seemed too simple, with death so very close. 'For the first time I saw it in front of me.' A friend of his, a writer he had known for many years and who was something of a confidant at this time, Dick Sharples, confirmed this: 'I got a phone call out of the blue, and it was Clive and I hadn't heard from him for a while so I asked him how he was, and he said, "Oh, not so good, I'm back in the Marsden," and then he started to cry on the phone, and I knew things must be serious, and then he said, "I'm frightened." So I drove straight over and he said, "This is it, they've told me I'm not going to make it through Christmas," and then he said, "I've never been frightened before but I am now, and I feel terribly alone," and then he asked me if I believed in God, in life after death, and I lied and I said I did. He needed that reassurance. So I tried to give him some comfort and some hope. But above all what I tried to give him was, if you like, anger. I told him to get bloody angry, to prove them wrong. I told him he'd done it before and he could do it again. Well he didn't just get through that Christmas did he? He got through two more after that.'

Clive underwent chemotherapy for the second (and last) time. Typically, the decision to go ahead with the treatment was not solely based on a wish not to face death just yet, but was partly made on rather coolly professional grounds. His play had been accepted by the BBC and was in fact in production and about to start rehearsals prior to being recorded shortly after Christmas. Naturally Clive wanted to see his play made, and that was what persuaded him in the last instance to have chemotherapy. He also asked the hospital to time the administration of the courses very carefully, so that neither they nor their inevitable after-effects would interfere with his ability to attend rehearsals or recording.

Actually the treatment itself proved to be less immediately harrowing and debilitating than he had thought it would be. The dosages he was given this time round were lower than in his previous bout, and the side-effects were, to his admitted surprise, less ghastly than they had been before. They were sufficiently wretched, however, for Clive to vow that he would never, under whatever circumstances, have chemotherapy again. He was continually vomiting or simply feeling enervatingly sick, and he could not eat or drink. On top of that, he was open to all manner of contagions, so he caught thrush in his throat, several bouts of flu, and a major urine infection. In addition, in order to strengthen him for the ordeal, he was on steroids, which bloated his face and his stomach, and unlike his previous bout of chemotherapy, although the dosages were lower, this treatment went on much longer, consisting of several courses of a week each once every six weeks – so Clive had to undergo several months of the treatment.

But it bought him the time to see his play made, and indeed to see it broadcast and to read the reviews it received and the hundreds of letters of appreciation, affection and encouragement that it spawned. Against all prediction, in fact, it bought him another two years of life and achievement. It is too easy to sensationalize this survival, to claim it as yet another 'victory' over cancer in defiance of both the disease and the doctors, as a further fine example of 'mind over matter', of the 'will to live' overcoming all. There can be no doubt that to some degree – and even his doctors and nurses will concede this – the fullness that was brought to his life by his sudden celebrity, and the 'purpose' he felt, largely as a result of the reactions to his play, did give him greater determination, a measure of 'fight', a certain anger – a 'rage against the dying of the light' – which contributed to keeping the tumour in abeyance; but this was always in tandem with the formidable contribution of medical science, the continual vigilance of the medical profession, and the careful administration of drugs.

The doctor responsible for the 'management' of Clive's illness and pain in the last four years of his life is prepared to concede, with caution, to there being a certain capacity of the mind to keep sickness at bay: 'I do know that the attitude and approach of some patients towards their illness can certainly and significantly influence how they cope both mentally and physically with the illness, and I'm sure in some cases that that attitude and approach can determine survival, within limits. I say that as someone who believes fundamentally in scientific medicine and who practises medicine on the basis of that belief.' He is insistent, understandably, that although Clive's mind and determination may have had something to do with it, what kept him going for the next two years was *primarily* that last lengthy bout of chemotherapy. When he was rushed to hospital nearly two years later in a near-comatose state, it marked another progression of the tumour into the base of the brain, an extension that would undoubtedly have occurred, and would have killed Clive, two years previously if he had not undergone chemotherapy at that time.

There can be little doubt, either, that Clive's emergence from that coma and his survival for another six months were also due *primarily* to extremely careful medical surveillance – or, as his doctor at the Marsden put it: 'He only survived because of the quality of the supportive care that he was getting, and the essence of that is the very high standard of nursing care that there is at the Marsden, the expertise of the nurses here in dealing with patients who are unconscious but who continue to need very potent drugs. The administration of such drugs under such conditions is a highly skilled business.' As he said these words I sensed the justified vexation of the expert in the face of ignorance, because the press of course chose to speak of Clive's recovery from his coma as a miracle and a triumph of the will – calling Clive a 'medical marvel' who had 'been defying the doctors ever since they told him years ago that his spinal tumour would kill him in months'.

In quieter and more private moments Clive would always acknowledge his debt to the Royal Marsden and to the friendly and honest care he received there, and he would express an appreciative affection for the doctors and nurses who treated him, even to the last. But the media attention he and his illness were being given once he had become 'a personality' made it quite difficult for these doctors and nurses to control his tumour properly because of a new tendency on his part to believe in his own legend; he felt he knew best and that he should indeed 'defy the doctors' by refusing to take their advice. This was all very well, and his privilege, except when it came to the dispensation of very powerful and complicated drugs, which of course had to be supervised carefully and accurately.

The Royal Marsden had always respected Clive's questioning spirit, his need to discuss, once his tumour had been diagnosed, every aspect of its development and how it was being treated ('He'd always have his little list of questions drawn up,' recalled Fiona Gardner, who was a nurse at the Marsden and became one of Clive's closest friends. 'He wasn't one of those who'd just sit quietly and say yes'), and the complex process of handling his illness was based on intelligent mutual regard, but in the latter stages of his treatment a certain distrust entered into his dealings with his doctors. It was a kind of reversion to his attitude to the profession in the years before the astrocytoma was found – and this made him, in medical terms, 'hard to manage'.

Fiona was forgiving of this behaviour: 'I think you have to realize that Clive had been through years and years of being pushed from doctor to doctor and being told that there was nothing wrong with him – and remember that he had a cancer that was difficult to get at, it was really hard to see how it was progressing, and his tests and his operations were always painful, always an ordeal – and you have to ask yourself if you've been through all that, whatever comes after that, are you really going to trust anyone ever again? Would *you* trust anyone ever again?'

Clive's truculence at the end was also the product of an arrogance that had always been a part of his nature, a healthy arrogance that in a sense was his own very special 'rage'. Although few people ever saw him angry, there was undeniably a kind of deep anger within him all the time, an anger which can also be called ambition. And while it is facile to talk of Clive's life as a 'triumph of the will', it is absolutely true to say that he died when his ambition died – when his anger went. 'Nearly each time Clive came into hospital,' Fiona recalled, 'he was always trying to get out. He had to be out by a certain date because something was going on, there was something to look forward to, something to keep his interest. That's how he kept himself going. And I think that in the last months he didn't really have that much to look forward to.'

It is arguable that it was the tumour that killed the ambition, because towards the end of his life it became monumentally difficult for Clive to achieve anything through sheer exhaustion. 'In the last six or nine months,' said Fiona, 'even when he was doing something he really wanted to do, it would take him one or two days to get ready for it, then two or three days to recover from it, so it became more and more difficult for him to stay interested in anything.'

Clive's final rage was a rage against living. His mother Maureen remembers his desperation to leave hospital: 'He kept saying, "Don't let them keep me here, don't let them make you keep me here," he was desperate.' His friend Elaine also remembers his need to get home: 'He said, "All I want is to go home." He said, "Promise me you'll speak to Maureen, and she won't let them change her mind, promise me you'll let me go home." I'd have carried him out of there myself if they'd said no, that's how I felt.' There were certainly efforts on the part of the Royal Marsden to make Clive stay, partly because it was the middle of the night, partly because he did need a blood transfusion before going anywhere, but also out of a genuine concern for those around Clive and the burdens they would have to bear ('A doctor took me aside,' Maureen remembered, 'and he told me, "You realize you're going to have your hands full." I said I knew'), but in the end they let him go. Clive had sensed a final medical conspiracy, which he interpreted in his desperation as scientific medicine's need to keep life going at all costs, and he was so very ready for death, so entirely resigned to letting the tumour win at last. 'When he got home,' Elaine recalled, 'he was smiling. He smiled for the first time in ages.'

3

AMBITION

ANTHONY Parker, a Light Entertainment producer at Thames Television, first met Clive in March 1980. 'I was directing an episode of *Shelley* and I was rehearsing on the studio floor, and it was getting close to lunch, when the floor manager tapped me on the shoulder and gave me an ear-piece to talk to the people up in the gallery and they said, "We've got security on the phone, and they say you've got guests," and I vaguely remembered that I'd arranged to meet a writer that lunchtime called Clive Jermain, so I said, "Yes, I'm expecting a writer called Clive Jermain", and they said, "Oh no, it's not him. Security know about him. This is a young kid who says he knows you, and he's got an old lady with him." So I asked them to ask security to get the kid's name, and sure enough his name was Clive Jermain.'

Tony had been telephoned a fortnight before by someone purporting to be a fairly established writer who was interested in writing television comedy. 'I thought the voice was odd, high-pitched, but I still thought he must be in his mid-twenties at least, because of what he was saying. I got this long speech about how good *Shelley* was, and that I must keep up the good work, and that there was an audience for that kind of programme. It was smooth flattering bullshit and I thought it was wonderful. So I let him come into the studio and meet me.'

Once it had been established that this 'kid' at the gate was indeed Clive, he was let through and taken to the studio, with his elderly female companion. 'I was getting on with things when through the corner of my eye I saw them drifting into the studio, brought in by the assistant floor manager – I saw this thin, very

69

pale young man, his hair very neatly combed, terribly frail. He had sticks, and callipers on his legs. He was walking quite well, swinging along, and he had a rather demure-looking old lady with him. She had a brimmed hat on, and a tweedy coat, a scarf and a handbag and those little old lady shoes. It really was bizarre. And I did have to wonder what my lunch was going to be like.'

He carried on directing, and the young man and the old woman sat patiently watching until the lunch-break. Then Tony went over to them. He saw that the young man was indeed considerably younger than he had assumed he would be, fourteen years old at the most. But he had a disturbing confidence and a quite aggressive manner. 'I'm Clive Jermain,' he said, adding instantly, 'You didn't expect me to be so young, did you?' Indicating the old woman with him he said: 'Can I introduce my nana?' Tony thought he might have said 'Can I introduce my nanny?' because he sounded, as Tony recalled, 'terribly well-spoken, upper-class'. On that day Clive did not bother to clarify that the woman was his maternal grandmother.

They moved towards the canteen, which was some distance from the studio. Because of Clive's disability it took them a while. 'The old lady hardly said a word, just smiled, and kept a few paces behind us all the time. As for Clive, I noticed those deep brown eyes flashing, taking in everything – absorb absorb absorb – and to be perfectly frank I found his behaviour a little disconcerting, because he was already – there's no other way of putting it – taking over.' It must have been not unlike escorting royalty, because Clive would stop and ask questions and would simply not move until he was ready, no matter how much urgency Tony was demonstrating (he had to be back and ready to start in the studio in an hour, and studio time is money). When they had made it to the canteen, and once they had settled down and started eating, Tony decided to be quite frank. 'Congratulations,' he said, 'you've really conned your way into the Light Entertainment Department of Thames Television,' at which Clive smiled a deceptively diffident smile and said 'It's not the first time, you know.' He admitted that he had not in fact written anything that had actually been shown on television, but added that he had every intention of doing so.

'As well as feeling a little annoyed at being so obviously conned,' Tony said, 'I did feel a sneaking admiration for the boy, as a working-class lad who's done his own bit of conning in his time. I've always appreciated that kind of tenacity, so there was immediately something about him that I didn't resent. And I can say honestly that I wasn't making allowances for his obvious disability. I remember accepting his disabled state and if I thought anything about it at all it was that maybe his tenacity and ambition arose from his incapacity.'

Clive and his grandmother watched the rest of the afternoon's rehearsals. At tea, Clive told Tony something about his disability – 'He said he had something wrong with his spine, and even spoke about a rod in his back.' At this stage there was as yet no talk of a tumour. 'But he did look terribly weak under his well-scrubbed appearance.' Then Clive said he had to go 'because he was tired', and as they were leaving the grandmother spoke substantially for the first time 'and even that was only a couple of sentences'. She thanked Tony and in her thanks, he remembered, 'I got the impression that she was very obviously quite proud of him but at the same time she was offering a veiled apology.'

Clive, of course, did not let this first encounter go by without asking if he could 'possibly let me look at some of his writing when he felt he'd got something for me to see'. Tony of course said yes – 'fully expecting the usual sort of stuff that ends up in a pile somewhere, unmade'. He confessed to a thought that is common among television producers: 'There's a selfish streak in all of us that tends to think with relief, "Well, that's him out of the way and maybe I won't hear from him again."' But no one in television whom Clive had made the effort to contact could entertain such misplaced relief for long.

'He behaved from that moment on as if I was now on a list of very special friends and privileged to be a part of that list. From then on there was no question that if he rang, I'd return the call, that if he wrote I'd reply. He expected it. And I felt a need to respond. Quite often the selfish side of me would think, "My God, he's taking over" – I'd be in rehearsals all morning and at lunch I'd ask the usual question, "Any calls?" and they'd reel off the list and then say, "And Clive Jermain wants you to ring him urgently," and it didn't seem urgent to me but I had to respect that it was urgent to him.'

Indeed, it was not the first time that Clive had gained entry to a television studio. He had even been to Thames Television before. At the age of eleven he had written to the company asking if he could visit the studios, and had received a polite refusal on the grounds of his age in connection with strict safety regulations. Not much later, as chance would have it, some of the cast and crew of a Thames Television programme called *Get Some In* happened to be drinking in a pub at which Clive's father was working at the time; contact was established largely through the father's persistence, and Clive was allowed to watch the programme being made on Sunday. 'So that was the first time I'd been in the studio. It was like a magical world to me, the only world I really wanted to be a part of from that early age.'

The studios which made even more of an impact were those at London Weekend Television on the South Bank of the Thames. 'It was something about that building, standing there all lit up. My mother was living in North London and I was living with my nan in Peckham, and every weekend we used to drive my mother home after she'd been to visit, and we always used to pass the London Weekend building.' When he was twelve, he recalled, he went with his grandmother to the dog racing at White City stadium. There were television cameras there, and Clive, typically forthright and unembarrassed, approached a London Weekend cameraman and asked him for his autograph. The cameraman, understandably flattered (it is not often, after all, that someone *behind* the camera is asked to sign an autograph book), had a conversation with Clive in which the boy spoke of his fascination for television cameras and studios – 'I think he was quite impressed by how much I knew about cameras. I told him how much better the L W T cameras were than the Thames cameras' – and it was not long before Clive was visiting the London Weekend studios. 'I was allowed into every studio they had. They were so good to me. Even on that first visit I was allowed to work a camera. And they gave me a London Weekend pass, which meant I could come back and get into the building whenever I wanted to.'

Clive took full advantage of his pass over the next few years, watching the making of something like eighty different programmes. 'I was allowed to operate cameras, booms, cables, and because all the crew members were willing to talk to me I learnt so much about the technical aspects of television production.'

From his earliest days, as far as he could recall, Clive's world was dominated by television. He was so much a child of his age – and perhaps of his class – that television was the well-spring from which all his thoughts, his desires, his pleasures flowed. It was only natural, therefore, that his ambition, like that of so many of his time, should have focused so intensely and from the very beginning on television as a profession, and ultimately as a means of achieving the celebrity he needed so consumingly.

He remembered other childish ambitions, of course. As a very small boy he wanted to be, somewhat oddly, a schoolteacher: 'I used to force my friends to be taught by me in the shed in our garden – I'd set it up as a schoolroom – and I'd stand in front of them and pretend to teach them.' Clearly there was a desire from an early age to dominate, to be in control, and to some extent to perform. He also subjected his obliging schoolfriends to quite detailed 'pretend' medical treatment when he harboured a thought that he might become a doctor – a not uncommon, though relevant objective, in the light of his subsequent history. In fact this particular ambition was still quite strong at the time of his early visits to various hospitals, during which his observant eye would pick up a few telling details which he would then take home with him: 'I used to give teddy bears drips. I got those bottles that you feed gerbils with, and fixed them to tubes from wine-making kits, and connected them to teddy bears. I used Ribena as blood.' But his predominant interest was always television and his overriding obsession was with a particular component in the making of television programmes – the most immediately apparent, in fact – the television camera itself.

It was a kind of mania. Clive himself remembered it as such. 'It was something about them. I think I just thought they were very beautiful – and as a matter of fact they were in those days, when they were much bigger.' He first saw a television camera on television itself, on a pop show called *Supersonic*. From then on he would watch television incessantly 'just in the hope of seeing a camera, especially the live programmes. I wrote a letter to ITN and suggested that at the end of the news they should pull back and show the cameras. I wrote another letter to Thames News asking the same thing. I bought all the books and annuals about television, only for the photographs of cameras.' It is not hard to imagine the thrill of enchantment that Clive must have felt when he first entered a television studio and at last saw these 'friendly beasts' at close quarters – or even better, when he was permitted to handle one.

Before this he had his own camera – an eight-millimetre Canon cine-camera, bought for him by his father from a photographic shop by Waterloo station for the very substantial sum of £90. Clive started to make films – some of them at home but for the most part at school, dragooning predominantly reluctant schoolmates into helping him as actors, lighting men, designers, sound assistants and general dogsbodies. He of course was always director and producer, writer and cameraman, and often star performer too. As a determined and domineering schoolboy, Clive had to be in charge. He had a 'best mate' who shared his enthusiasm, helped him write the scripts, designed sets, and acted too, but the rest of his friends rarely had sufficient patience to hang around the set for long, much to Clive's annoyance. They found it hard to tolerate the boy's obsessive need for perfection in all things – his insistence on 'going for another take' when the first take was not technically acceptable 'because the microphone was in shot'. Even at this early age Clive was 'trying to do it properly, professionally'.

There was a good deal of role-playing involved too. 'Playing the part' of being a director, or writer, or cameraman was every bit as important as, if not more so than, the finished product. The films were always meticulously scripted – 'It was never just a case of "going out there with a camera".' Great effort went into the layout of the scripts, naturally enough, so that they would have a suitably 'professional' appearance, even down to the command at the bottom of the front page: THIS SCRIPT IS THE PROPERTY OF CJP AND NO COPYING IS ALOUD.

CJP was 'Clive Jermain Pictures'. We have all been guilty of self-important games of this kind when young, and although they may seem childishly silly with hindsight, there is no doubt that out of such vagaries genuine skill and dedication can emerge. Clive himself retained no illusions in later years about the films he had made when he was young. They were, he readily confessed, 'terrible' – usually little more than a string of ill-connected slapstick antics, and gags culled from every joke-book available to him and his friends. Television was invariably their basis; television programmes were referred to, television personalities were portrayed. However embarrassingly schoolboyish they were, though, there is no belittling Clive's dedication to them at the time.

The output of CJP was prodigious, and the preoccupation lasted three years, until he was thirteen. The last film Clive and his friends made, a substantial epic called *The Zany Show*, was made during the summer holiday and cost all of £100. It was no better in content than its many predecessors, only longer and more expensive. Shortly after this holiday, Clive was admitted to hospital for his spinal fusion. There was to be no more film-making after that.

Film as a medium never interested Clive, then or subsequently. He was wholly unfashionable in that sense. He got through three film cameras during his short and boyish 'film-making career', and it was typical that the camera for which he had a marked preference was the one that was least efficient but which 'looked like a television camera because it had two humps on the back'. The fact that it kept breaking down did not seem to matter. Its appearance was far more important than its efficiency, and what was most important to Clive was his function in the whole business and the involvement of a camera that he could pretend was a television camera. He remembered how at the age of about eleven or twelve he would, with the usual careful attention to detail, set up a news studio in his bedroom at home and pretend to read the news to whichever of the cameras he possessed at the time.

'I'd put my white projector screen up and sit in front of it, put on my tie-clip microphone, set the camera up in front of me, facing me, and read the news. When I had more time in the day, during school holidays, I would buy all the newspapers and edit the stories, changing their order of importance until the last minute, then at one o'clock I'd switch my little tape recorder on and it would play the one o'clock news music, and I'd read the news.' It was a performance entirely for his own benefit. No one watched him, only the silent, filmless, non-functioning camera. As the years passed he would involve other people as the fantasy became more sophisticated, employing members of his family and even obliging neighbours to act as his 'team', who would hand him last-minute items 'on air'.

Shortly before he went into hospital for the operation on his spine, Clive appeared briefly in front of real television cameras, as a 'guest presenter' on one episode of a Saturday morning children's programme called *Our Show*. It was a small break obtained through his contacts with London Weekend Television. He was immediately disquieted by the comparative self-assurance of his youthful co-presenters. One boy, who is now quite a well-known young actor, particularly impressed him: 'He had it, the professional quality. He could be sulky, moody, just an ordinary boy when the cameras were off him, then as soon as he was on camera he became bright, smiling, sharp, in control. The transformation was brilliant.' Clive's appearance on television turned him into something of a star at his school – 'They all watched the programme and some got rather jealous.'

He had endeavoured to appear on television before – auditioning, unsuccessfully, for the children's show *Crackerjack*, applying for an audition for *Opportunity Knocks*. So he had a wish for stardom of a kind, in a wider world than that of his school (or his home, where as his grandmother's darling he would give little 'shows' for her benefit, cracking jokes, doing 'impressions'), from quite an early age. He also had a predilection for bombarding television companies with letters of one sort or another, only really to make them acknowledge his existence. These were often, curiously, letters of complaint, usually about bad language. There were also the inevitable requests for photographs and autographs, several further endeavours to get into television studios other than those belonging to Thames and London Weekend, and letters asking for advice as to how to become all the things that Clive then wanted to become – a cameraman, a director, a producer, a writer, an actor. 'Dear Master Jermain,' the Head of Drama at Yorkshire Television wrote. 'Thank you very much for your letter asking how to become an actor. I must tell you that it is a very hard profession as I know because I was an actor once but I am not one any more. The best thing for you to do would be to stay on at school and try to get as many O and A-levels as you can . . .'

When he was only ten Clive sent off his first script, to a producer at Thames Television. It was called *Danger Children* and was about two boys running away from school who were kidnapped by a group of villains who they discovered were trying to assassinate the Prime Minister. The script was four pages long. The producer returned it with a tactful reply: 'Thank you for letting me see your script. It was very exciting if a little short. I am sure it will be fun for you to make when you get your cine-camera, but in all honesty I can't see Thames Television ever making it . . . Keep plugging away and one day you might be doing my job.' It was three years before Clive sent a revised, longer and more mature version of the same story, now called *Escape and Kidnapped*, to other producers in other television companies, who sent encouraging if inevitably guarded replies. The script was of course very juvenile, in form as well as content, but it nevertheless showed promise – a promise so youthful and unformed that it was impossible to tell if it would ever be fulfilled. But the Head of Drama at ATV, David Reid, told Clive that he was 'very impressed' and that his story-telling ability was 'excellent'.

This was after Clive had had his spinal operation and had returned to school 'very behind in my work and feeling a bit left out'. The rough and tumble of school, in which he had participated with enthusiasm in spite of his pain and a certain incapacity, was now forbidden him. Inevitably he became more thoughtful and introspective – and perhaps, if only subconsciously, aware of the possibility of a hampered future. He recalled that it was at this stage that he made a concrete decision 'to become a writer'. He had read an article in a magazine about a girl of his own age who had won a prize for a television play which was actually going to be made, 'And I suppose I thought if she can do it so can I.'

It was entirely typical of Clive that he thought he could 'become' a writer, just as he could 'become' anything else he might turn his mind to, and that all that was required was the decision. A year or so previously he had written to Dick Sharples, the writer who had conceived the ATV series *General Hospital*, and who was now its script editor, with an idea for an episode about his own ailment, curvature of the spine. Dick Sharples remembered receiving the usual flattering letter 'telling me he was an avid watcher of the series and how he'd always admired it, and how he wanted to be a script writer and he knew we hadn't done a story on scoliosis, which he knew about because he had it'. Dick had sent back a polite rejection, telling Clive that it did indeed seem a good idea but regrettably the next season of the series was fully commissioned, 'And I told him to keep writing, and not to be upset by rejection, that I could paper my living-room with the rejection slips I got before I managed to sell a script.' Clive now chose to renew his contact directly by calling in on Dick without warning in his office at the ATV studios at Elstree in Hertfordshire. 'I went up to the desk and asked for Dick Sharples.' As it happened he was out of the office that day, 'But they rather foolishly and improperly gave me his home phone number.'

Dick was by this time no longer working on *General Hospital* but on a new series which was set, ironically, in a children's ward. As Dick recalled it: 'Clive rang me and the next thing I knew I'd invited him up to the studio to meet the cast with the producer's full approval, and that was it.' A strong friendship was formed that lasted the rest of Clive's life – it was one of several such relationships (like that with Tony Parker, which began a year later, or with the cameraman George Cann, who was to become his godfather), between bluff, perhaps cynical, seasoned professionals and a young boy whose only desire was to be famous on television.

Clive unarguably wove a kind of spell. Dick Sharples said that 'He definitely had an Oliver Twist quality about him, but behind that mask there was maturity.' His effect on people naturally had something to do with his disability and the sympathy it compulsively evoked, but it was primarily born out of his wholly unapologetic, and always charming, persistence. It is not an injustice to remember Clive as a very manipulative young man. Dick Sharples said of him: 'His inventiveness in developing relationships without giving offence was quite remarkable. He was never on the defensive, never apologetic, which is a lesson one usually learns much later in life. One learns that being apologetic embarrasses people and that one diminishes oneself by saying "sorry for being so much trouble". Clive was *never* sorry for being so much trouble.' He had the very ambitious person's ability to make those important to him feel flattered that they should be considered so important. 'His cleverness,' Dick said, 'was that everyone he contacted was made to feel that it was only that person he'd contacted. He made you think that he had one or two very good friends but that you were rather special. Everyone was a best friend.'

Such views of Clive are based on profound affection, because he was never malicious in his manipulation of people, and also on admiration for the manner in which he controlled his short life. He was indeed in charge of his destiny, despite the pain, and the fear, and the frustrating incapacity. As Dick recollected: 'More than any other person I know, Clive made his own luck. *He managed his own life marvellously.*'

The management of his life around television and its opportunities continued intensively after he emerged from his first long bout of hospitalization. An encouraging response to his *Escape and Kidnapped* script from Tyne Tees Television prompted a visit to their studios in Newcastle, where Clive was asked to submit ideas for the children's show *Check it Out*. As it was International Year of the Disabled, Clive decided to do a taped interview with a young spina bifida patient he had befriended in hospital ('The irony was considerable, looking back on it, asking a boy what it was like to be stuck in a wheelchair'). Nothing came from the idea but it showed that, as he had already demonstrated by sending the scoliosis idea to Dick Sharples, he was becoming aware of the uniqueness of his medical situation and that it might be used to his professional advantage. There was still a part of him, though, that wanted to be a comic. As soon as he had met Tony Parker at Thames, he inundated him with scripts of and ideas for comedy sketches and situation comedy episodes. He was not afraid to mention his medical state in the many letters that accompanied these submissions, from the very beginning:

> I have been having trouble with my back and the rod, which is inside. My doctor said that the fusion, which is meant to be straight, is not and is thus putting pressure on my kidneys and the whole of my right side. Also an abcess has formed at the top of my spine! Anyway I've got to go and see the surgeon and see what's going to happen soon so maybe he'll be able to put me out of my pain. Anyway before my problems started again I managed to finish three sketches . . .

The problem with all the scripts and ideas that were sent in was that, as Tony Parker readily admitted, 'they simply weren't funny'. The second-hand, slightly smutty, schoolboy humour was still very present.

At school itself Clive remained mentally, if not quite so physically, active. There were no films, but he edited the school magazine and wrote a play with an extremely serious and notably mature subject – teenage alchoholism. He researched it in some depth, attending meetings of the teenage branch of Alcoholics Anonymous. Clive could still not think of himself solely as a writer – in writing a play about a young alcoholic he was writing a part for himself to perform. The play was never put on. At fourteen he left a school that he had learnt to enjoy and went to one he hated. It was too 'sporty' for his taste. Nevertheless he edited a magazine there too, and started to promote the idea of forming a school film club, or of using film more generally as a means of broadening the school's Arts curriculum. The love of cameras was still strong. In fact the combination of this love and a thorough distaste for his new school led him to play truant quite frequently, and to spend those illicit hours in the studios of London Weekend Television.

It was London Weekend that gave Clive his first substantial writing commission. Humphrey Barclay, the Head of Light Entertainment, paid Clive to write a half-hour pilot for a children's comedy series. Clive worked hard on several drafts, but before there was any chance of perfecting the episode to the point of his being satisfied with it enough to deliver it, he had to go into hospital again. He was fifteen and he was going to have his tumour removed. This hospitalization put an end to his schooling too.

Clive's creative life and the pursuance of fame understandably suffered something of a slowdown during the next two years. His mental and emotional energy had to be channelled into the effort of coming to terms with the sudden onset of paralysis, then with the news that the paralysis would be permanent, and finally with the knowledge that he could not be expected to live much longer. On a more fundamental level, there was the enervation of the treatment and the exhaustion of physiotherapy, and the opportunities to be creative were in any case limited by his continuous hospitalization. Also, religion dominated his thoughts to the exclusion of much else. For a palpable period of time, ambition, television, celebrity must have seemed monumentally irrelevant. Furthermore, it is very difficult for the mind to be properly and happily creative when it is hampered by feelings of bitterness, and there is no doubt that Clive became severely bitter for a while – a propensity that he did not reveal to any but those closest to him. It must have been a peculiarly impotent bitterness too, based on a general but deep sense of injustice but with no one in particular to blame. It was unequivocally a black time.

Slowly, strongly – and it must have involved a colossal effort of will – he pulled himself out of the blackness and started to write again. He was seventeen. The first thing he wrote was a situation comedy which he sent to various producers – a curious piece about a boy living with his grandmother, which were Clive's circumstances at the time, an odd mixture of autobiography and wish-fulfilment (the boy is continually trying to escape his grandmother's rather puritanical clutches) – too close to his own experience to have the objectivity of true comedy, too fantastical to be convincing, and again, simply not funny enough.

Reactions to the script were polite but non-committal. Then Clive let the more serious side of his mind take over. It was a kind of liberation. He wrote a short play for television that for the first time concentrated on putting across what he felt about things rather than on trying to make people laugh – possibly he was beginning to sense that making your grandmother and your close relatives and friends laugh is the easiest thing in the world compared to coaxing laughter out of strangers. The play he wrote, called *One of the Boys*, was still not terribly good but it was super-abundantly better, because generally more honest, than anything he had written before. It was about two school friends – one bookish, the other sporty – who meet up again after some years; the envy of the studious boy, who is also encumbered with diabetes, for the liberated, sexually active athleticism of the other leads to murder. Although much of it was set in a hospital, Clive was not yet brave enough to use his own situation fully. But the play – in actual fact more of an idea than a play – was informed, unquestionably, by Clive's own feelings of impairment, inadequacy, and loneliness.

It may not have been a wonderful play, and no one would ever have produced it, but it was written out of heartbreak. When I read it (Clive sent it to me on the advice of David Reid, who had responded so inspiringly to *Escape and Kidnapped* four years previously), I knew nothing of Clive's plight, only that he was young. I recognized at once the feel of youthful, slightly rough, semi-auto-biography, because I myself had written a few undisciplined screams in my youth, but I fear that I gave it insufficient regard at the time, considering it a reasonably accomplished example of teenage angst. I responded with the reserved encouragement that I would offer to any young writer who demonstrated a degree of promise.

Clive also sent his play to the director of the television serialization of *Brideshead Revisited*, Charles Sturridge, whose response was no doubt more inspiring than mine: 'I thought it was extraordinarily well thought out and presented with a good sense of pace and a real feeling for film . . . I sincerely hope that you do not find this . . . letter discouraging, the assurance with which you write leads me to believe that this will not be the case. So be brave, be original, and say what you think . . .'

This last advice was the very best that could have been given to Clive, for he still had a clogging concern for form over content. There was still so much a part of him that was playing the role of being a writer as opposed to simply writing. Something of the old love for the way a script 'looked', the way it was laid out, was continuing to hamper him – a concern for the neat spacing that he had learnt from studying hundreds of camera scripts, for the pedantically detailed stage directions, so specific that they even described the pattern on a character's tie or the colour of his toothbrush. The things that should have come last – if indeed they should have concerned him at all – seemed to come first. What was prevented from emerging properly as a result was what Clive thought and what he felt. There was of course no clear evidence of the true anguish of his existence. If there had been I should have wanted to meet him immediately. As it was, I did not do so for well over a year, during which time he wrote a play into which he poured his whole tortured being.

In October 1983, when Clive was eighteen, he wrote to Tony Parker:

When I left Stoke Mandeville, I felt, physically and mentally, fitter than I had done for some years. After another operation to fuse the spine the pain was much more bearable, though still present. My life as a result was transformed. My writing was much more fluent, being able to sit up longer to type. I have finished one single play, was sorting through two ideas that I had for a situation comedy and had just started on another single play. Then my world was devastated. My nan, whom you know, was taken into hospital and diagnosed to have a tumour at the back of her throat. Now, so ironically, she is in the same hospital as I was, going through the same treatment as she saw and helped me through just over a year ago! To me, my nan has been an unfailing support and constant source of encouragement always. So life seems to be dealing out some very severe blows and I have not felt like writing anything, even putting off letters, and wonder whether I'll ever feel like writing again. My nan has a great deal ahead of her to cope with, as I know only too well, but she is very determined, and I know she will make a full recovery. Life for me, unfortunately, is very much like a sea-saw, up one day, down the next. The pain has returned and dictates what sort of day I will have. My mind, though, is still very active with thoughts and ideas, which in many ways is frustrating because I am unable to get them down on paper. However, I do so hope that we can keep in touch and that I will not be forgotten . . .

Shortly after writing this letter, Clive had to undergo his first ever bout of chemotherapy, and then his grandmother died. He had started to write the 'other single play', which was *The Best Years of Your Life*, just before his grandmother was admitted to hospital. 'I researched and wrote most of it while she was in the Marsden,' he recalled. 'I felt guilty about that, I didn't feel I was giving her enough time, but another bit of me knew she'd understand, that it was what she wanted. She was the only one in my family who ever really encouraged me in my writing. Not that she ever read anything I wrote! But she believed I wanted to to do it, and believed I should do what I wanted to do.' The chemotherapy impaired his creativity for a while, as did the shock of his grandmother's death, and coming to terms with the loss of her presence and constant support, but not for long. He had in effect 'completed' the play by the summer of 1984. In Clive's terms, it had been 'a long haul', taking him about eight months.

Talking about the play to various interviewers, Clive liked to say that it was his grandmother's death, allied to the knowledge of the imminence of his own, that had given him his ambition, which he called a desire to 'achieve something for which I'll be remembered'. Experiencing the way in which the world seemed to go on after his grandmother had died, he said, had made him determined not to be similarly ignored. But this narrative of his creative life should have given the fairly clear impression by now that Clive's ambition was a fundamental facet of his nature long before he was made aware of his mortality, of the terrible tentativeness of his existence – unless there is indeed something in the doomed one's subconscious that makes him sense the brevity of his life long before he is certain of it; as was perhaps the case with Keats, Clive's favourite poet. Possibly it was not just coincidence that Keats *was* Clive's favourite poet – or that his favourite Keats poem, first encountered when he was fourteen, before he

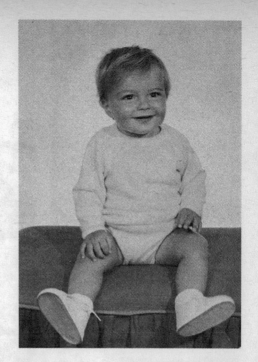

Clive's childhood.

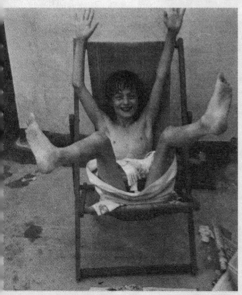

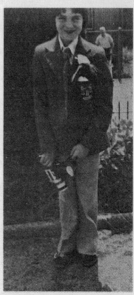

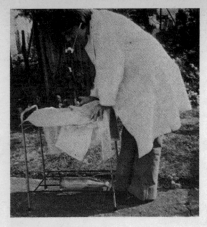

An early ambition.

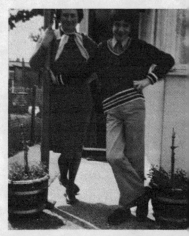

With his Nan outside the prefab.

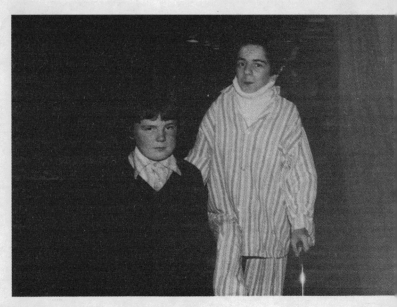

With younger brother Lee shortly after the rod was put in.

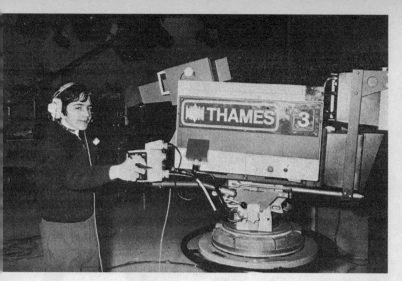

At Thames Television.

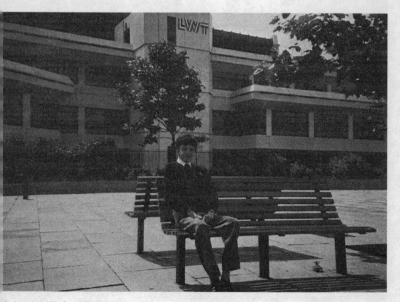

At London Weekend Television.

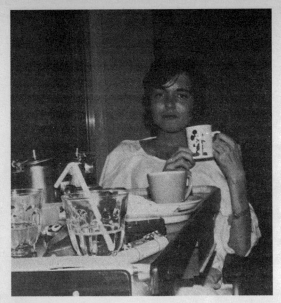

During radiotherapy.

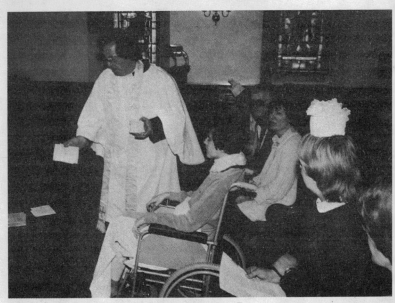

Being christened and confirmed in the Royal Marsden Chapel.

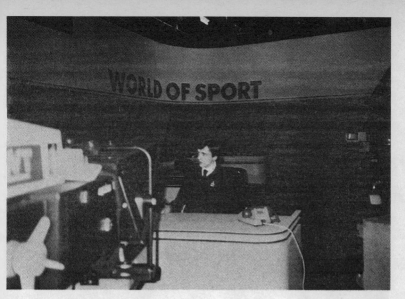

In the *World of Sport* studio.

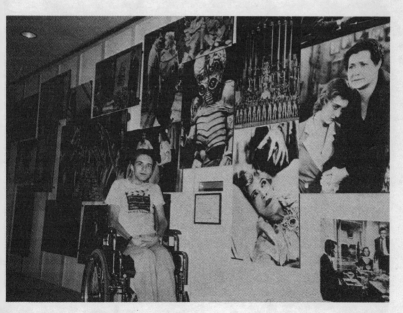

In Hollywood.

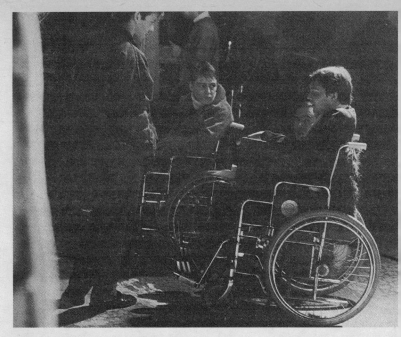

In the studio for *The Best Years of Your Life* with, left to right: Steve Fletcher, Lee Whitlock and Stephen Kramer. (BBC)

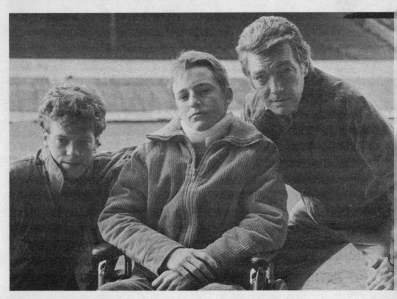

The Best Years of Your Life: Steve Fletcher (Mark), Lee Whitlock (Robert) and Alan Ford (father). (BBC)

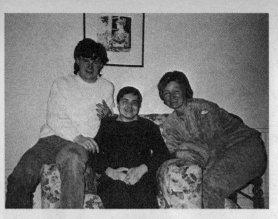

With Lee and Maureen on the night of the play's transmission – 14 May 1986.

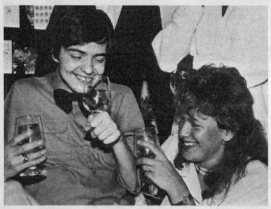

With Fiona on his twenty-first birthday.

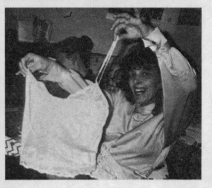

Elaine with a Christmas present.

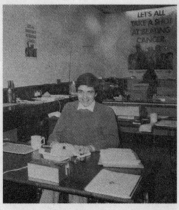

In the Search '88 offices, Soho Square.

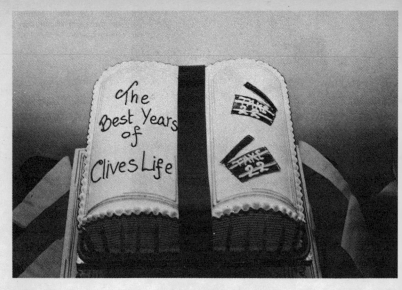

The last birthday cake.

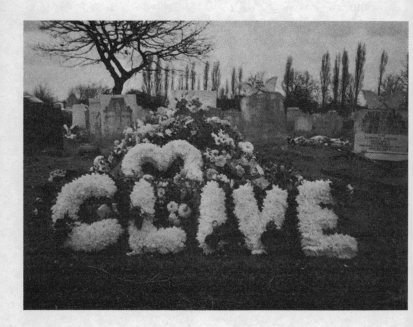

knew he had a tumour, was 'When I Have Fears . . .'. Neither, perhaps, is it simply coincidental that a line in an essay Clive wrote when he was twelve was picked out by his English master as being particularly striking and demonstrated certain intimations of impending death and a life beyond. The essay was about a garden and the line was: 'The leaves fell to the ground and lay dead, resurrected by the next wind.' All this is very uncertain. What *is* certain is that Clive himself liked to pinpoint these associations as examples of his having lived a rather Keats-like life himself, for he was very capable of a degree of self-dramatization (and who could begrudge it him?). What is equally certain is that Clive was not Keats, although he sometimes liked to think he was (and who could begrudge him that either?).

Clive sent his play round to the usual assortment of possibly interested parties, including an agent who was prepared to represent him on the basis of it, and to Charles Sturridge once more, who considered it 'an enormous development . . . funny, shocking and moving', but who had to admit that he could do nothing with it because of other commitments. He asked Clive to telephone him, and he mentioned various other people who might be interested, including me. As Clive waited for a response, he pursued his partiality for comedy again and managed to obtain a commission to write the warm-up routine for the comedian Jim Davidson on one episode of the comedy series *Up the Elephant and Round the Castle*. The series was produced by Tony Parker, who admitted that he commissioned Clive 'more as a favour to the boy than anything else'. Clive was paid £200, and duly wrote a monologue that lasted about two minutes. The monologue that was actually performed was rewritten so completely by another writer that only one of Clive's gags remained. But typically what mattered more to Clive was that Tony's 'favour' had included a screen credit – his first as a writer.

Clive also fulfilled another long-cherished ambition at this time – he visited Hollywood. He paid for himself and a 'minder' from the Spinal Injuries Association. 'He had to get a bank loan,' his mother recalled. 'It took him about a year to pay back.' The trip lasted three weeks, and was enormously exciting (he had never been abroad before, let alone to California). Privileged treatment (they were picked up at the airport by a stretch limousine with a black chauffeur) was ensured by contacts in the film and television industry back in England, including the film producer David Puttnam, to whom Clive had written unabashedly explaining his situation and his outlook and saying that he had a dream of seeing Hollywood before he died.

Another television executive involved with the arrangements recalled that Clive was in no way sheepish about his illness, his disability, or the fact that he did not have long to live when it came to obtaining what he wanted. The entire visit, she recollected, was organized as a kind of favour to a dying boy – 'He lived for another four years as it happened, but then it was as if he only had another five minutes.' To Clive's delight, Hollywood was no longer the world's *film* capital, but a place where many of the American 'imports' he had seen on television were made, some of which he now watched being filmed. He also took a few copies of *The Best Years of Your Life* with him, 'just in case I ran into an important producer'.

On his return from America Clive drafted a letter to London Weekend Television asking for a job. He never sent it, perhaps because it sounded simply too agonizingly pleading. It had a real desperation – the entreaty of a young man seeing the end of his life approaching with awful rapidity:

I have experienced . . . changes in my body and great pain. I have been diagnosed as having a tumour in the spinal canal. After an unsuccessful operation to remove the tumour I was left in a wheelchair. All that I knew had been totally turned upside down and I left hospital to face a shattered world. All through my illness my friends at L W T have been a constant support, comfort and encouraegment, through times of great depression and frustration. I do not tell you this to gain your sympathy, but to try and convey a deep sense of urgency. I desperately want to do something for L W T before it is too late. Although I am disabled I feel that I have a great deal to offer. My interest would be working in presentation and promotion. The job I would like to do is continuity announcing, which I could do regardless of my disability. I think I have a good voice and a smart dress sense.

The precise nature of the fame that Clive craved in his ap-
prehension did not much matter – what mattered was fame at all
costs, and as soon as possible. He *still* could not think of himself
solely as a writer. Even in less frantic moments he was still considering how fame might be achieved through other avenues
apart from creative writing. He was extremely keen, for instance,
to be an actor, and one of the motives behind writing *The Best
Years of Your Life* was his hope that he might play the leading
part himself. It had been the predominant purpose in the compo-
sition of a play at school about a young alcoholic, and he had not
yet grown out of that dream. At around this time, too, he conceived an idea for a documentary series about young people,
called *The Youth Today*, for which he prepared a very detailed, if
slightly unfocused, treatment which he sent to London Weekend
and other television companies.

It is notably ironic that the means by which Clive did at last
achieve the fame he had pursued so tirelessly since the age of ten
should arrive on my desk at the BBC without even a hint as to
his medical circumstances – when he had so recently had no
qualms about putting a tragic and highly emotive situation at the
service of his ambition. Perhaps this said something about Clive's
opinion of the work in question – that he did sense that it was
something that was so very much more important than anything
else he had previously created, and that as such it needed to be
taken very seriously indeed, and considered on its own merits,
without any special pleading. Clive himself liked to give the impression, when talking about the play, that he had never accorded
it any very great significance, that he had not been able to see in
it anything that set it apart from everything else he had written,
at least not when writing it, and it is of course very often the case
that the writer is the last to notice the depths in his work. Clive
insisted to the very end that what he had *set out* to write was 'a
play about football, or at least about a young footballer who
suddenly couldn't play football any more, and had to come to
terms with that'. The fact that the young footballer had cancer,
and died of it, seemed to be of less consequence to Clive than the
fact that he was disabled. 'I wasn't going to give him a tumour at
first. I was going to make him have a car accident. But a tumour

was what I had, and I knew about it, and if he had a tumour, he had to die really, didn't he?'

Clive's somewhat phlegmatic attitude to his hero's death was an indication of how he felt at this stage of his life about the imminence of his own – he could not consider the boy's death in the play as being tragic, or even sad, at least not for the boy, because he could not see his own impending death as either of those things, at least not for him. Death, to Clive, at the time of writing *The Best Years of Your Life*, was nothing but a 'welcome release' (his preferred way of describing it) – from the pain and the frustration of his disability. And so it was to his hero.

But in spite of Clive's adamant protestations as to the modesty of his intentions when creating the play, what he in fact wrote was only marginally about football, or disability – and it was indeed about death, and love (those two irresistible stalwarts), and if it had only been about what Clive claimed he wanted it to be about, it would not have attracted my interest (or anyone else's, I suggest) sufficiently to get it made. I also think that Clive knew, while writing the play, even if only subliminally, that what he was creating was important because it was truer to his feelings and longings than anything he had created before. He certainly knew its worth, and acknowledged it, once the play had come out.

When I received *The Best Years of Your Life* I was a script editor at the BBC with recently-born ambitions to become a producer. I can state with certain hindsight now that my own ambition at the time was a prime factor in ensuring the realization of Clive's wish to see a play of his on television. This is not a boast, only a suggestion that the travail and exhaustion involved in getting the play made and transmitted might well have made a less hungry producer buckle under and abandon the fight. I had nothing else to go to. I needed a project. The play's director, Adrian Shergold, joined the struggle for a not dissimilar reason nearly a year after I first reacted to Clive's play. He had already directed some distinguished work for television, but he had reached the stage in a relatively green career when he too needed something special with which to make an assured mark, and he recognized this opportunity at once in Clive's play. I make this point to emphasize that neither of us were in the business of doing anyone any favours. We saw in Clive and what he had written a chance for ourselves. I venture to suggest that for Clive and his play this was a good thing, because we were not prepared to vacillate or weaken in our determination to make the thing good.

That said, it took me a time to react positively to the script as it stood when Clive sent it to me in the autumn of 1984. Because I knew nothing of Clive's circumstances, I did not immediately put it 'at the top of the pile'. When I did read it I found it hard work. It was rambling, wildly disorganized, and extremely long. If it had been made as written in that first draft, which would never have happened, it would have lasted well over two hours. It was full of dross and unnecessary detail. I could not recognize at the time that what Clive had done was simply to 'put it all down', obeying the instructions to 'be brave . . . and say what you think', without, at last, undue attention to the niggling demands of the writer's craft. Much of it, as a result, was simply tedious. But something shone through for all this, and it held me in the end. I was drawn by the simplicity and heartbreaking directness of the fundamental story (and the story is always the great test).

The play is about a boy of seventeen who lives in a small South London flat with his father and his elder brother. The mother is dead. The brothers have a friendly relationship based on jovial small-talk. The father barely says a word. They muddle along. The boy has ambitions to be a professional footballer – he's good, he's played for the Chelsea youth team, the Apprentices. The twist is that he has cancer – a growing spinal tumour which is not only going to kill him eventually but which, because of mishap during an exploratory operation, has paralysed him and confined him to a wheelchair. It is a devastating affliction which forces not only the boy but also his father and his brother to examine themselves and their feelings for each other, to pull themselves out of their separateness. The two boys declare their love for one another; the father is about to do the same, in his own way – but the boy dies before he can.

If there was any one part of the play that rendered it distinctive in my experience it was the single scene in which the two brothers said they loved each other, something which they had never done before, but which now, overriding their initial boyish embarrassment, they knew they had to do, because otherwise the one would die without the assurance of the other's love. In a first draft that was still in many places over sentimental, this scene, which should have been the most sentimental of all, was somehow the least, because it came across as being vibrantly true, even at this early stage. Although I could not yet be certain of it, the reason for this was simple – it was written from the heart. The scene, and because of it the play, was Clive's own cry for love.

As the script waited to be read and reacted to on my desk and was then read, re-read, and considered, Clive was jotting down his appallingly sad fears and desires in a very personal collection of writings which he started about this time – there were not many, but they all make stark reading – which he liked to call his 'thoughts':

The past few days have been dreadful. The pain has been so very bad accompanied by some breathing difficulty and now a near-continual sickness. I've been going around crying, not knowing what to do. Mentally, I still feel that I want to do so much, to write down all the ideas I have in my head. To make the longing even more frustrating I received a copy of 'What's New at LWT' this morning, full of news of their new programmes, some completed, some in planning stages . . . Trying to get a job at LWT might soon be unrealistic as for the past few weeks I've been seeing things slowly getting worse; the pain, the sickness, not being able to sit up straight, being generally much weaker, especially upper limbs – even sorting through my photos the other day tired my arms! *I want to write so much, but every time I try to type my ideas out the pain gets so bad.* It is very frightening . . . slowly, almost subtly, losing another piece of movement, suddenly realizing: 'I could do that a couple of weeks ago . . .' Since I've been back from America I've lost so much. Oh, I am so frightened, because although I welcome death as a great release, I fear the bit towards the end – slowly getting worse and having to rely on somebody else for more and more. I only hope that it's not too long and drawn out like poor nan. My only hope now is that I can achieve my few remaining ambitions before I die. They are, above all, to have my play THE BEST YEARS OF YOUR LIFE filmed, and to take the leading role, to write a sit-com, a screenplay and another two plays, have a good Christmas *out of hosp*, go to LA one more time, and be the subject of 'This is Your Life', which I'd always told nan I would be . . .

A belated Christmas present arrived in early January 1985 in the form of a telephone call which, unknown to me, brought a timely rush of optimism to Clive's life. As far as I was concerned, all I was doing was ringing Clive up to tell him that I had enjoyed his script and considered it to have great potential, and would he like to come in to the BBC for lunch with me and my then producer, Brenda Reid?

There was never a moment when Clive told me, or when I was told by anyone else, that he had cancer, or when I myself asked the crucial question. He assumed that I would assume that that was what he had when we first met, and to a certain extent I did. Here was a boy in a wheelchair, after all, who had written about a boy in a wheelchair, and the boy he had written about was dying of cancer, so surely the similarity between protagonist and author had to be taken to its logical conclusion. But there were also certain crucial differences between Clive and Robert, his hero, the most immediately apparent of which was that Robert was a streetwise South London seventeen-year-old with a passion for football, whereas his creator seemed to be a very tidily presented, delicate, well-spoken young man of nineteen who, as he confessed at our very first meeting, had known nothing about football until he had to research it for the play. So possibly I was not being wholly obtuse in not making an immediately convinced connection between Robert's illness and Clive's. He did, I recall very vividly, look ill, behind what I sensed to be a thoroughly prepared exterior – he had slicked-down black hair, and a general scrubbed sheen to him. I was to see him much iller, but on first acquaintance I could make no comparisons and in a sheltered life I had never before been so close to such obviously serious ill-health. Nevertheless for some reason, possibly squeamishness, my own response to the cancer taboo, I could not be absolutely sure that Clive had cancer until I rang him some months later, after we had met several times, to arrange yet another script-meeting, and he told me that he could not see me at his home but that we would have to meet at the Royal Marsden Hospital.

Clive was to confess to me when he knew me much better that he had in fact taken hardly anything in during that first meeting with Brenda Reid and myself. He had been entirely overwhelmed by the thought that his play might actually be made. He was also trying very hard to be relaxed enough to listen to what was being said to him. He told me too that before leaving home for the appointment he had been violently sick – literally sick with fear – and that this happened prior to several further meetings. For most of his life Clive had to make extraordinary efforts to overcome the pain and sickness and anxiety and panic that dominated his private existence so as to present to the world a collected, calm, confident 'public face'. As it happened, there was little for him to absorb at our first encounter, except our enthusiasm and encouragement. He had occasion to wonder, though, during the full year it took to get his play recorded, if he had not been somewhat misled by our initial excitement, if our 'seriousness' about the play had been genuine. He wrote about his feelings in his 'thoughts':

> I suppose it was because I was a new writer. Everyone kept saying how good it was, but still there was such a delay. I really began to question whether they were telling me the truth. Was it that good? If it was why wasn't someone doing it? David kept telling me it wasn't just a play, it was an event. I didn't know what he meant.

Clive was giving vent to what was very much a standard feeling of writer's paranoia, except that in his case of course there was an added urgency that made him very different from the average writer. And as he waited, and patiently rewrote draft after draft of the play in order to satisfy our continued demands for improvement, his health did not stop declining, the pain and the impairment of course continued, and he alternated between despair and sad hope:

I got a copy of 'What's New at LWT'. On the first page was news that Melvyn Bragg was planning a series for Channel 4 called 'Great Writers'. That really hit hard, making me realize that I would never be considered among the great writers. People will undoubtedly say 'oh he was very young'. But look at John Keats, who died in his twenties, look at how prolific he was and how much of life he experienced! I have noticed that as well as the pain stopping me from writing, apathy has also set in. I don't seem to have the mental strength. I find my mind wanders all the time. I notice that I tire more quickly and am very weak. I see these writers turn out play after play, series after series, and wish, wish . . . I pray, at the moment, that God may push and motivate me to finish the rewrites to my play and that I may be fit enough and pain free enough to take the role of Robert, which I would be pleased to be my epitaph. I pray that it may be God's will too.

Clive was not to know it, just as we did not always appreciate his own anxieties as fully as we perhaps should have done, but we were battling for his play, and it was a tough struggle. The script was indeed very rough through several drafts, and the improvements that Clive was making were understandably slow in coming through and sometimes when they did come through they were minimal. But in my view we were always moving, however slowly, towards something extraordinary. The longer the fight continued, though, the more it seemed the powers above us needed to be convinced.

Ironically, when the full truth of Clive's situation was known to all concerned, the difficulties were not eased but compounded. The more we talked of urgency, of Clive's illness and his possibly extremely imminent death, the more we were accused of letting our knowledge of Clive's condition cloud our opinion of his work, and of asking for the go-ahead to make this still rather unpolished and perhaps somewhat juvenile play simply as a favour to its dying author, and not because it was a good play in its own right. I would respond adamantly that my judgement was being mistrusted, and that I had been moved by the script before I knew it was semi-autobiographical. I added that I did not as yet think it was an especially good script technically, but it was getting better all the time, and that it would be exceptional. Clearly we were not going to be allowed to give Clive the assurance that his play would be made until it *was* exceptional. Tempers became frayed. All the time we were telephoning Clive, or writing to him, or visiting him at his home or at the Royal Marsden, to endeavour to keep some optimism going – 'I sometimes thought,' said Clive, 'that if this is writing you can keep it.'

Brenda Reid said that if I could get the green light to make the play I could produce it, and she went off to work on other things. With the freedom at last to be in complete control I quickly set about getting a director interested who could then, if he liked the play sufficiently, or saw potential in it, fight for it with me. I asked Adrian Shergold to read it and told him that it was written by a nineteen-year-old boy who was dying of cancer. He read it immediately and was at once enormously affected by it. He said something that I had not really thought about before but which suddenly seemed obvious: 'The boy's written about his own death. He's written his own death into a play.' He said that for that brave reason alone he wanted to direct it.

Within a few days of making this decision Adrian was visiting Clive regularly and talking to him about his life and his illness. Much of what he gleaned from Clive during these conversations ended up in the play. Clive told him, for instance, about how many pills he had to take – at that time eight pills every four hours – and Adrian rightly pointed out to him that that was something people should perhaps know about and that there should be some reference to it in the play, or better still a scene in which Robert is seen to be taking the pills and has to explain to his brother what each pill does. Clive took some persuading as to the effectiveness of such a scene because to him of course the pill-taking was a very routine feature of his own life and therefore, in his opinion, merely boring. There were also aspects of his illness and his disability which for understandable reasons he preferred not to have to mention or even think about too often, and we had to convince him that the more distressing such matters were to him the more important it became to make people aware of them. We were trying to give him the courage to face up fully to his own situation – something which he still was not quite doing – because only by facing it completely could he convey the truth of it to others. He was still occasionally hiding behind sentimentality and false emotion, and we were determined to rid the play of all traces of mawkishness.

In the late autumn of 1985 two things happened almost simultaneously: first, we obtained permission to make the play subject to a few further script changes, to Clive's considerable relief and delight; and second, Clive quickly suffered a huge deterioration in his health. He was told that he would probably not see his play made unless he was prepared to undergo a second course of chemotherapy. Horrible though he knew the treatment would be, he decided to endure it, with every expectation of dying soon after the play had been recorded. He was also, therefore, facing, for the first time, the terrible closeness of death.

Within a short while of being given the agreement in principle to go into production with the play, and having even reached the point of casting some of it, we were suddenly told that, on the basis of the script as it stood – although it had changed substantially since we had received the go-ahead – we could not continue. We could not inform Clive of this new blow – not in the state he was in – so we embarked on a fairly desperate ploy which in retrospect saved his play. We went home and over one weekend we took the play apart and put it back together again, cutting, sharpening, reshaping, and 'toughening it up' generally. It was something which I am sure we could have achieved with Clive in time, but time was what we and (as far as we knew) Clive did not have.

As we waited for a reaction to the new script, Adrian and I went to a party at Clive's flat. He was out of hospital briefly in between bouts of chemotherapy and had decided to throw a pre-Christmas 'thank-you' party for all the people who had helped him in achieving his ambitions so far. The local bakers had prepared a rectangular cake for the occasion on the top of which was written, as on the front page og a camera script:

'THE BEST YEARS OF YOUR LIFE by Clive Jermain. PRODUCER David Snodin DIRECTOR Adrian Shergold, BBC TV, Mcmlxxxvi.'

Clive made a speech before cutting the cake, reeling off a list of thank-yous. Everyone apart from two of the people mentioned on the top of the cake assumed that the long battle to get Clive's play made had been won and that the waiting was over. It was hardly a pleasant moment for us as we sat with fixed smiles receiving Clive's gratitude. He looked ill, desperately wan (although the full effects of the chemotherapy had not as yet made themselves felt) – but for the moment he was happy.

On the basis of the final rewrites the project was on again. Only when we were absolutely certain that it was no longer under threat did we bring Clive in to explain what we had had to do and why we had felt that we could not in the circumstances have burdened him with the problem at the time. To this day I cannot be sure how happy Clive was with what we had done to his script – he chose never to tell me. Typically, he understood the situation and that we had had no alternative, in that his play would not have been made if we had left it as it was, and what mattered to him, as always, was that the play should be made. In any case he did not have the time – or the energy then – to be excessively sensitive about his work.

We gave him the rewritten script and asked him to take it to another office in Television Centre and to read it there and then. We offered him the opportunity to be as angry and obstructive as he wished, to 'throw the script out of the window' and demand that the three of us sit down and start all over again, if that was what he wanted – although I have no idea what we could have done if that had occurred. He took about two hours to read the script. When he had finished, he said nothing but the word 'fine'. He accepted it wholly as it stood. He did not look best pleased – but he also looked exhausted and resigned. The script he had just read was the script that was made. I postulate that for all the cuts and additions and shifts of emphasis that it had undergone since it first arrived on my desk it was still Clive's play, born of his unique experience and forged by his feelings, his fears, his wishes, his disappointments, his inner anger, and his intense need for love. Whatever Clive thought of what we had done, he got his revenge – if revenge it was – when a version of the play was staged at a London fringe theatre about a year and a half after it was first televised. Much of what we had excised was put back in.

AMBITION

The Best Years of Your Life was recorded in January 1986. Clive did not of course play the leading part as he had rather fondly hoped he might. On medical grounds alone it would have been impossible, as he was extremely weak because of the chemotherapy, and he understood this, but he would never in any event have been allowed to play his hero. As it happened he made his wishes apparent when it was too late – the part was on the point of being offered to the actor who eventually played Robert – but we would never have contemplated the possibility anyway. We were not, as I have already made clear, in the business of doing any favours.

Clive was extremely disappointed. His friend Fiona Gardner said: 'It was a very strong desire right up to the point when he had the chemotherapy. It was the one big aim in his life, writing the play and being in it, but he soon realized it couldn't be that way . . . but being aware and accepting are different.' For a young man with such a craving for fame it must have been exceedingly crushing to have to reject an aspiration held for so long. In his 'thoughts' he wrote:

> Day in day out, I practised my South London accent, going through my lines – playing Robert, to me, was the most important thing. Then I became very ill, deteriorating very rapidly. I was in enormous pain and taken into hospital. I was told what I really knew, that there had been some progression into the brain stem. Although I could be put on steroids, it could only be for a short time, the real choice was whether or not to have more chemotherapy. The thought of more treatment filled me with dread, but everything was on the line, my play being produced and me thinking that I could probably play the part . . . This is the major reason I wrote 'The Best Years', tailored for my needs. In retrospect, it is the biggest regret of my life . . . I was simply too scared to audition . . . like most things in my life I left it and I left it . . .

There was some solace in his recognition of the extraordinary and accomplished sadness of Lee Whitlock's performance as Robert.

In fact he was for the most part entirely enthralled by the

process of production, so much so that it often made him forget the vexations of his sickness – so acute at this time – and indeed his pain. No one involved in the play can forget the sight of him on a freezing January night at Stamford Bridge, Chelsea Football Club's ground, white-faced and wide-eyed, wrapped so completely in blankets and scarves that only the top of his face could be seen, and refusing to be wheeled into the warm until the night's work was over. It was only when he got home very late that night that he realized he had forgotten to take two of his four-hourly doses of diamorphine – in other words, he had felt no pain for eight hours. His absorption was similar on a blisteringly windy night by the side of the canal – 'My mum and my brother were so cold and bored that they disappeared indoors pretty quickly. But I wasn't going to budge however cold I got. I know it can get very boring when all you're doing is watching – there seems to be so much hanging around when nothing is happening – but I wasn't bored for a second!'

If he did start to find the business tedious and begin to feel a touch ignored it was towards the end of shooting when the pressures of time imbued everyone, as is always the case, with a self-absorbed sense of crisis. He wrote: 'So many people seemed so involved, performing their particular jobs, I did feel very left out . . .' More than once I caught sight of him sitting quietly and a little morosely in a dark corner of the television studio, the only one with nothing to do. Occasionally a friendly cameraman would allow him to sit behind a camera that was not being used. At the small end-of-recording party, when fond farewells were said, he seemed terribly bewildered, clearly unable to accept that it was all over. A lot of people did not know that he was returning to reality at its cruellest – two days later he resumed his chemotherapy.

The play had been made after a year of dashed hopes and anticipation and anxiety that I would not wish on any writer, least of all Clive, but our battles were not quite over. The next struggle was to get the piece transmitted while he was still alive. Now the play was made it became exceedingly important to Clive that he should live to see it on television. He wanted fame so voraciously that the entire process had to be experienced, from inception to transmission and the glory that he hoped would be the result. He liked to speak nobly of 'leaving something behind', and to a great extent that was what he wished, but he also wanted to be talked about and applauded, to be 'important', *before* he died. It was a need for instant adoration, born I think out of loneliness, that at times could make his innermost longings and unhappiness seem self-pitying:

> Yesterday was a fantastic day. I went to the BBC TV Centre to watch the play again, this time with the cast . . . As we drove up to the gates the adrenalin started to pump . . . and once again I felt important. Lee, Zoe, Steve, Wayne and I went up to David's office. David and Adrian and Alan Ford were waiting. David's office is small and we crammed in. Whether it was not hearing but Adrian . . . seemed to ignore me. We all went up to a 'conference room' where David opened bottles of champagne. The play was shown. The end credits rolled and as Producer came up everyone clapped, as they did again for the Director, but no applause for the writer!

As far as Adrian and I knew, Clive had a few weeks to live after the play had been made, possibly a couple of months at most. We were not alone in thinking this; it was the general prognosis. Transmission was scheduled for the summer of 1986, by which time we genuinely thought that, barring a miracle, Clive would be dead. None of our entreaties on his behalf seemed to move anyone into altering the transmission date. We were not being entirely altruistic in our efforts. No producer or director likes his programme to go out in the summer, when the evenings are light and the general theory is that it will not be given the attention it deserves.

We managed to arrange a screening of the play at the British Academy of Film and Television Arts, as a 'favour' to Clive, so that at the very least he could enjoy some kind of reaction from people other than those closely involved with him and his play. Again we were also doing it as a favour to ourselves, in that we sent invitations to most of the significant film and television producers in the country, an extraordinary number of whom turned up, for Clive's sake. A sprinkling of 'celebrities' also came, to give the occasion a degree of glamour. We had asked Clive if there was anybody famous that he most particularly wanted to meet, and he at once mentioned the actress Joanna Lumley. She was invited, she came, and was so moved that she gave Clive a gold bracelet with her name on it, there and then. It was obviously an item that meant a great deal to her, and Clive's mother Maureen wears it now.

Clive made the decision to undergo another bout of chemotherapy the day after the BAFTA showing, to give himself a further chance of seeing his play on television, but he was not going to allow that close prospect to cast a shadow over this, 'his night'. The screening theatre was packed, and the play's effect on the audience was immediately apparent. People were enormously, visibly moved. The most pleasing aspect of the evening was that the play *had* seemed to work on its own merits. That was the view expressed over and over again. Clive was in his element – the absolute centre of attention, being congratulated by the important and the famous. I had never before seen him so openly happy. He treated himself and a clutch of relatives and friends to a 'Dinner at the Ritz' after the showing. As he left the BAFTA building I thought he looked positively well – not tired, or even pale, but actually glowing, it seemed, with achievement.

4

FAME

As a result of the showing of *The Best Years of Your Life* at the British Academy of Film and Television Arts, at which certain selected journalists were present, as well as some significant people in the television industry who made a point of mentioning the play and Clive's situation to their friends in the BBC hierarchy, the play was suddenly scheduled to be shown on television only a matter of weeks later. The primary determinant was undoubtedly an article in *The Times*, which began: 'TO ACHIEVE AND THEN TO DIE. Clive Jermain is 20. He is articulate, bright – and dying of a tumour. He hopes to live long enough to see the play he has written televised.' It ended: 'The play is still waiting for a transmission date. On Monday it was shown at the British Academy of Film and Television Arts. On Tuesday Clive went into the Royal Marsden for a third course of chemotherapy to keep him going because he wants to see his play broadcast.' It was a lengthy, intelligent and considered piece, telling Clive's story directly and movingly. At its centre was a large photograph of Clive himself – a head and shoulders shot, the wheelchair out of sight. It could have been the picture of a healthy, bright-eyed, amiable young man, an anomaly which lent greater poignancy to the sad tenor of the article itself.

More newspaper articles were soon to follow. The play received an exceptional amount of publicity for a fifty-minute drama on BBC-2. Clive's condition was of course eminently newsworthy. Gaining the media's interest involved virtually no effort at all, for his story was one that sold itself. On the whole it was treated gently and responsibly. The *News of the World*'s headline –

CANCER BOY'S REAL LIFE SAGA – was a touch bald, especially for a young man who himself still found it hard to use the word 'cancer' when describing his medical situation, preferring to refer to it as 'a tumour in the spinal canal', as that did not seem to have such an immediately deadly ring to it. Clive's attitude to his illness progressively hardened as the publicity it received intensified and continued beyond the play through his other achievements in the two years left to him, but at first it was very difficult to have to face up to his circumstances being forced upon him so very publicly. 'There was a period when you couldn't look at a paper that didn't have a picture of me with *cancer* written beside it.' He explained his discomfiture in a documentary about him that was based on a series of interviews with Adrian Shergold:

> . . . I still find it incredibly difficult to talk about. And . . . when . . . reporters were saying, 'Well, what's your condition?' and, 'Do you know how long you've got?' . . . I found that terribly difficult to answer. And also it was very much a shock to me to actually see things in print like 'Clive Jermain, who has spinal cancer' . . . It's rather like reading about a private part of your life which you've almost in a way . . . hidden or covered up . . . I suddenly thought about how my mum and close friends and relatives would take it. And I suddenly thought about it the other day as well, when we were . . . rewinding the tape of the news and really it was a bit like watching a favourite movie over again. But the message in it was a very serious one, and here were newsreaders . . saying, 'And the play . . has been written by a twenty-year-old man who is dying of cancer' and we were sort of watching these tapes over and over again as if it were . . some favourite film. And I . . . wondered about what sort of impact that must have had on my mum . . . you know, to keep hearing about the illness. It was . . . like somebody really reinforcing what had been said once, and which you only want to hear once really . . . suddenly there it was, either on the television or in print, the full realities . . .

Clive was becoming famous very quickly, which was something he had always longed for, but now, on first contact with attention outside his immediate circle, he was not sure that he was being made famous for the right reason. He undoubtedly wanted to be in the public eye, but perhaps not for having cancer. His disability, too, was something he did not particularly wish to be known for, not at first. He still considered it an embarrassment, a stigma.

The previews that the play received were extremely encouraging. *The Guardian* called it 'beautiful'; *Time Out* said it was 'outstandingly good'; the *Sunday Times* described it as 'a work of great distinction'; the London *Standard* said that it was 'intensely moving to watch, firstly because it is very well-written ... secondly because its author has the same dread affliction. Though the work is not autobiographical, Clive Jermain has been able to tint his play with the kind of detail that can be drawn only from a deep, dark well of experience. A poignant, powerful piece – not easy viewing but one from which it is well-nigh impossible to turn away.' On the day of transmission Clive appeared on BBC *Breakfast Time*, then he was interviewed for the lunchtime news. The same item appeared on the six o'clock news and even on the main news at nine o'clock on BBC-1, only minutes before the play itself was due to start on BBC-2. Clive watched the play over dinner at my flat, with his brother Lee and his mother, who had missed the BAFTA showing because she had been abroad:

> I had no great feeling watching it go out as not only had I seen it before but I had been writing it for a year and a half. The only feeling I did have was of embarrassment watching it with my mum, wondering what she was thinking. After all, I was doing it to be immortalized. I'd have much preferred to have been talking on the news about what it felt like to be the youngest director employed by the BBC or something like that, but the story was my situation. I also said a lot of things in the play I could never have ... discussed with her.

The next morning every paper carried a review and all were enthusiastic. *The Guardian* called the play 'a fine drama début'; 'a powerful piece, completely clear and alive', wrote the *Daily Mirror*; the *Daily Telegraph* wrote of 'scenes as poignant as an audience could take'; and *The Times* said that 'this portrait of stoical resignation punctuated by spurts of emotion rang absolutely true'. The Sunday papers continued the praise. The *Sunday Telegraph* considered the play 'almost unbearably moving' and 'an overwhelming triumph for its young author'. The *Mail on Sunday* wrote: 'The script was a sequence of brief, clean, under-stated scenes, the dialogue was terse yet pin-sharp, without a redundant syllable ... Emphasis was held back, and the pure poignancy flowed through. It was heartbreaking.'

The importance of such notices, to Clive and to all those in-volved, was that none was being simply kind. If they did mention Clive's circumstances, they were careful to point out that the play was fine by any standards, which was the most gratifying response Clive could have wished for. But what was to have a more profound effect on him, to the extent of changing his attitude to his own situation, was the response he received from the often-so-silent public: 'After a few days of calm, the letters started. The first day it was one medium sized BBC envelope. There were about fifty letters in it. The letters continued. Every day a BBC envelope arrived, with many many more letters.' He received something like 400 letters as a direct result of the transmission of his play – a quite exceptional reaction to a television drama, as Clive himself acknowledged: 'It's quite often you see something on television and you think it's so good that you want to write to someone about it, but you don't get round to doing it, because in the end it seems an effort. But all these people made the effort.'

Because there was no indication in his play that his hero held any specific religious belief, only the vaguely expressed feeling that there 'must be something more', many of the letters that Clive received were urgent assurances of the 'good news' that God existed. 'I have good news for you, Clive,' so many of them said, as if by rote. 'God exists and He loves us so much that He sent Jesus Christ to us to suffer for us.' Some of the exhortations were more than a little forthright: 'Do you realize you are going to MEET GOD, and are your sins forgiven?' To the more contemplative letters in this vein Clive replied personally, but there were so many that he could not respond to them all individually, so he sent a patient pro-forma reply: 'I am glad to say that I already have a very strong faith, which has been of great help and comfort to me during my illness and many difficulties during my life.'

Clive never forced his faith on anyone, which was a sign of its strength. He never once thought of referring to it in his play. He considered evangelism irrelevant and frankly embarrassing. He was therefore more profoundly affected by the letters that were free of the entreaties to 'find God before it is too late', and which simply told him what a very good play he had written, and how moving it was, or to what extent it related to something in the letter-writer's own experience. Some of these were very touching indeed, indicating to Clive 'how much pain there is out there', and he could not but feel spiritually proud of his powers of communication when he read letters from people who had found his play a comfort and a support in their own suffering.

There were also, of course, a good many cranky letters, offering any number of remedies for his illness. Many of the letters were from people close to his own age, including a schoolgirl who wrote, with unintentional bluntness and to Clive's great amusement, that she hoped he was not dead by the time he received her letter! A letter from a woman in her eighties told him to hurry up and write his second play, as she was herself dying of cancer and wanted to see it before she died. Out of the several hundred responses, the one that seemed to stir him most was from a medical student of whom Clive wrote in his 'thoughts':

> He said that he had just joined medical school, but was not certain which field he wanted to work in. After watching the play he wanted to devote his life to researching and treating cancer. He thanked me for guiding the course of his life! WOW!!!

But the main impression that Clive received from the letters *en masse*, '90 per cent of which came from people who had never been in contact with cancer', was the feeling of a need for further enlightenment, and a desire to make some greater contribution to the fight – 'they wanted to know and understand more about it, as well as *do something*'.

Without doubt such a huge reaction filled Clive with a 'sense of purpose' that he had never felt before. It was a very profound change. It made him wonder if he was quite ready for death, when there now seemed to be something to do. He would have found the word 'mission' somewhat grandiose – and indeed it is in his case, because however worthy his achievements, every one was motivated at least in part, and often the greater part, by the overwhelming wish to be famous – but the fact he suddenly found a function in life which seemed to indicate a purpose behind all that he had endured cannot be questioned:

> During my illness I'd been given books written by people who had overcome or were coping with great tragedies in their lives, but through their faith had found a 'purpose'. Despite my faith I had never been able to see a purpose – why a relatively active young man should be turned into a 'living carcass on wheels', which is how I saw myself for a very long time. I was forever told that 'God worked through weak people', and that He had given me the ability to write. Even that I could not accept, because although you could say that I was given that ability it seemed useless, because it was overpowered by my pain, and my disability, and the endless problems, hospitalizations, treatments, operations, infections. So it seemed that although these people had problems they were nowhere near what I had to go through, every day and every night. However, now, for the first time in my life and during my whole illness I could see a reason why – a point to it all. I remember just praising the Lord and thanking him, thanking him for using me and for helping me to see the point . . . I felt really inspired, especially spiritually. I desperately wanted to do something . . . I wanted to do something that would immortalize my name and me . . .

The 'purposelessness' of his life had led him prior to this to talk of death as a 'welcome release'. He would speak of Robert's death in the play in these terms, and it was for this reason that he could not, while writing the play, think of it as being an especially 'sad' end to the story. Clive's referring to death as a 'welcome release' was rather hypothetical and related to his faith. When he first faced death as a very real prospect, shortly before his chemotherapy, he was terrified, and had to revise his opinions. But after the play's broadcast and the response to it he did not so much fear death as shun it, in the 'not quite yet' sense: 'I started thinking "not yet" after the reaction to the play, with all the letters, and the enjoyment of it, and after years of hassling people to give me jobs and take an interest in me I suddenly got people writing to me and phoning me up and saying "would you do this" and "would you do that" – it suddenly all seemed very worth it, and worth going on.'

Having written a play about cancer, too, seemed 'worth it' in a way it had never seemed to be while writing it or while it was being made. He now sensed the play's true 'purpose'. Having created something that he modestly claimed was inspired by nothing more than 'a sudden interest in sporting ability' and thoughts as to what it might be like not to be able to play football any more – and a story in which the fact that his hero had cancer had seemed to be of marginal import – he saw the good that had come out of his being honest about himself and his own condition. 'I didn't think it'd be any help, honestly, to push the cancer thing, but the letters made me realize it had helped people, so there was a reason behind it after all.' He found a purpose in his play and a purpose in his suffering – genuinely – and death, 'the welcome release', would have to wait until more had been achieved. If this could ensure further appearances on television, all the better. 'As it becomes more of a reality, the closer it gets, the more you say, "Well maybe not yet, well maybe I'm not quite ready for it, not just yet, maybe there's just one more thing to do, then I'll be ready, but not yet."'

The new 'sense of purpose' also allowed him to accept the idea of his condition as a public phenomenon. The young man who had winced at being called a 'cancer boy', who had always wanted to be famous but not because he was in a wheelchair and about to die soon, at last recognized that he stood little chance of becoming famous for anything else, and with his newly-discovered vocational zeal (allied to his driving need, as always, to be on television at whatever price), he now saw no reason to be particularly unhappy about this inevitability. In the two years of his life after the play was first broadcast he appeared on television with some regularity, but always in association with his illness or his paralysis or both – because of his involvement with the cancer venture Search 88, or as one of the presenters on a programme about disability called One in Four.

His substantially researched and immaculately presented treatments for further television programmes, none of which saw the light of day, were all unashamedly related to his state – a major documentary series about cancer, an arts series aimed specifically at the disabled viewer, a clever documentary called *The Media and Disability*, which challenged the able-bodied viewer's preconceptions about the disabled and which began with Clive himself reading the news as an apparently 'normal' presenter, after which the camera would pull out to reveal that he was sitting in a wheelchair. It was an interesting reflection of Clive's continuing opportunism that it had to be *him* sitting reading the news, something he had always wanted to do since the time he had sat in his bedroom doing just that in front of his cine-camera. As Fiona Gardner said, the ultimate ambition, however nobly motivated otherwise, was always 'to be on the screen, as whatever, as an actor, as himself, right up to the end basically'.

The aspiration to be a newsreader was incidentally one that he would quite probably have fulfilled if it had been his fate to live longer. Martyn Lewis, the newsreader he got to know through their mutual interest in Search 88, is convinced of it: 'He'd be sitting where I sit now, in a matter of a few years. I'd have had to look out for my job.' Chris Hutchins, the producer of *One in Four*, is also certain: 'He'd soon have been doing something like *John Craven's Newsround*, the news for young viewers, then working his way to the nine o'clock news.' He indubitably had the ability to be immediately and absolutely assured on camera – a talent he had admired in a co-presenter on the children's programme *Our Show* when he was still very young, and which is rarer than one might at first assume.

Referring to a future that never occurred begs the question as to how his writing might have developed. Dick Sharples considered the first scripts Clive showed him, when he was about fifteen, as 'very promising for a young man who would probably make it eventually'. Had he been in a position to do so, he would most definitely have commissioned something from Clive, and not just 'as a favour'. He was at the time running a series which required the expertise of highly experienced television writers, but 'Had I been running a series of new plays, say, with a brief to encourage new writing, I'd have had him in and I'd have worked with him on a play.'

Teenage promise is a hard thing to judge, unless it is patently brilliant. It can so easily never develop further than that first demonstration of potential. On no account should it ever be discouraged, of course. But even I, who worked with him on his writing more exhaustively than anyone else, cannot say for certain that I know how Clive's talent would have progressed. It would be dishonest to claim, simply to be kind to his memory, that he would assuredly have become a fine writer. But he might well have become one. It is impossible to tell on the basis of the one fine play he produced, not only because of the hard graft and the many rewrites it took to make it fine, but because it was, from the very start, such a personal and unique piece – written from the heart and from within a singular experience. It was a one-off through circumstance, and could have remained so had circumstance been different.

The worn adage comes to mind about it not being the first play, or novel, that is the hard one to write, but the second. It is true that Clive found it achingly difficult to think of what to write after *The Best Years of Your Life*, and he so very much wanted to write another play. He came to me with a few ideas – the most interesting of which was called *The Care Attendant*, about the relationship between a disabled young man and his 'carer'. It was not dissimilar in theme to the play he had written before *The Best Years*, in that it was about the envy of an incapacitated person for a 'normal' one. Clive could not make it 'get anywhere beyond the basic idea', so we dropped it.

Adrian and I had what we thought might be a good concept to think about – a young man in a wheelchair with a video-camera, an obsessive film-maker, is pushed around London by his grandmother, who also stars in the film he is making, together with whoever might be passing by. We suggested to Clive that he research the play by going round London himself. He could borrow Adrian's video-camera and just film and talk to anyone who happened to be around. He could have famous people as the 'passers-by'. Clive tried to take to the notion, but in the end he could not, probably because, although based on his own experience and obsessions, it was not his own. In any case, he often insisted, what he *really* wanted to write was something that had nothing to do with cancer or with disability. But Clive's experience of life did not go beyond his illness and his incapacity, and he was too young and immature, in essence, to write about a world other than the one he knew.

The severe case of 'writer's block' that Clive endured from the time he finished *The Best Years* until his death only applied to original, fictional writing, which he knew only too well is the hardest writing of all. It was compounded by his illness, by the crippling weakness from which he suffered in any case, by the increasing number of days in any one week when he could do nothing but be ill. That he achieved what he did in the last two years of his life is remarkable and humbling in any event, and there was no shortage of 'projects' for him to devote himself to – all of them involving considerable time and energy, and a good deal of 'writing' in the form of very detailed treatments. Clive's imaginative writing stopped, in effect (apart from a few random 'thoughts' and the occasional snippet of poetry), not much more than a year after the first broadcast of his play. He did not appear to be especially unhappy about this. The 'sense of purpose' that he found because of the reactions to *The Best Years* had by this time taken him down so many other fulfilling avenues. I still think, however – and of course I can be accused of bias – that the time of writing and making his play was the most creatively and professionally happy period of his life. I am sure that Clive recognized an unequivocal achievement in himself for a brief while then as he was never to do again – something within him that was important and enduring.

Clive was thrown into the world of fund-raising and 'good works' in a small way before he knew it was happening to him. Within two weeks of the play's broadcast, he was taking part in a 'fun-run' for the *Sport Aid* appeal for Ethiopia, wearing, like everyone else, his 'I Ran the World' T-shirt. He had been drawn into it because another guest of BBC *Breakfast Time* on the morning of the play's transmission had been Bob Geldof, the organizer of the *Live Aid* concerts and record, who, according to Clive, 'told the world I'd be taking part before I'd said I would'. But he enjoyed the event, which to his great pleasure was televised, and it made him think more about charity work, most specifically in the field that related directly to his own situation.

'Although I was talked into it, I soon realized how important it was. And with the letters I thought God has suddenly shown me what he wants of me, and he's suddenly using me. I suddenly got that feeling. And with the run for Ethiopia that Sunday, I realized that I could actually use the publicity I had got, for whatever reason I'd got it, actually not just to gain better understanding of what cancer-victims were going through, but perhaps actually to raise money for cancer, and then to help in other ways, to help people understand, perhaps through making documentaries.'

It was not long before Clive was thinking of some form of televised cancer 'event', of which he would be the inspirational centre. His thoughts were immediately large-scale. He had neither the time or the desire for small beginnings from which greater things might grow. The exorbitant nature of his plans also had something to do, indisputably, with the proliferation of enormously ambitious charitable events at that time, of which *Sport Aid* was one. Indeed, this powerfully prevalent fashion for extravaganzas organized around a whole variety of noble causes rendered it inevitable that someone else apart from Clive should be conceiving of an event concerned with cancer almost simultaneously – as he was to discover to his great disappointment soon enough. To begin with, however, the energy and sheer hard work he put into organizing and selling his concept of a television-based 'Cancer Week' – set, he initially thought, for May 1987, the anniversary of the broadcast of his play – were extraordinary.

What started out as something called 'Action Week Against Cancer' became, predictably, 'Clive Jermain's Cancer Week' ('something to immortalize my name and me'). People other than Clive became involved, and helped him formulate and express his ideas for what was to be the longest 'telethon' yet broadcast – a whole week of programmes related to cancer, including a repeat of his play, naturally, and the documentary that he knew was being made about him by Adrian Shergold and another director, plus a major series of documentaries about cancer in general, for which he wrote precisely and thoroughly researched, and indeed impressive, treatments. The series was to be called *The Big C*. There would be televised fund-raising efforts throughout the week up and down the country, with the inevitable array of stars and personalities. There would be a *Live Aid*-inspired 'charity pop gala'. Other concepts bubbled up with a fertility born of increasing enthusiasm. Although no one concerned had any experience of working in the minefield of charitable institutions, cancer charities were approached by Clive and his friends, and they expressed a degree of interest. The BBC seemed interested too, although only informally.

Clive came to see me in my office at the BBC after a meeting with the then Controller of BBC-1, Michael Grade, at which he had talked about his project. I had not been in contact with him for some months – nor, till then, did I know anything about his Cancer Week. Describing it to me now, he seemed energetic, fervent, happy. There was an obvious zeal in him that I had never met before. I was surprised, because this was the young man who was now supposed to be dead, whose play we had fought to have broadcast earlier than originally scheduled for that reason. I wished him luck because what he was conceiving sounded undeniably exciting, but I was forced to wonder silently if such a frail figure could possibly have the strength, or finally the will, to bring such a monumental project to fruition. Certainly he would not have been able to do it in the year he had given himself to make it happen, at least not on such a scale. But he had the right combination of ambition and noble purpose now to make something along those lines occur at some stage, if he was allowed to live long enough, and if he was given the right kind of support. 'I was happy and I really thought it could happen. But it didn't get anywhere because of ignorance really.' He wrote in his 'thoughts':

I was convinced that the week had to be on a major scale, nationwide, because like everything you only get one chance. We had such good ideas, but ideas were what they stayed as. There were so many hurdles and questions that we just did not know the answers to, nor did we know the people who could answer them. But we pressed on and got the support of many celebrities, who gave us interesting contacts and even a personal message wishing us luck from Mrs Thatcher.

Matters were really quite well advanced, therefore, when Clive learnt by telephoning an acquaintance at the charity Cancer Relief that someone else was planning a large-scale series of cancer 'events' of some sort, not for the following year but for 1988, which had been designated as Cancer Year. What was being created in fact was a new and highly ambitious initiative to raise money for the cancer charities, called Search 88, 'And they were already so much further ahead than we were.' When Clive asked the acquaintance from whom he had received this body-blow to tell him more about what Search 88 was planning, 'She rattled off a list of their activities and support, which was like being blasted by a machine gun.' Then she asked him if he wanted to meet the man behind the new venture, and Clive of course said yes.

The telephone call immediately plunged him into deep depression, predictably, for the simple reason that it now looked as if someone had stolen his thunder. He buoyed himself up, however, by considering the possibility of a merger with the impressive-sounding Search 88, and he still clung to the concept of a Cancer Week in his name, but now as part of their activities. Perhaps, he thought, the week could act as something of a 'prelude' to all that they were planning.

Clive described Gareth Pyne-James, the prime mover behind Search 88, as a 'very blunt South African businessman', but he sensed 'behind the arrogant exterior . . . a kind-hearted man'. Even on first contact over the telephone it was obvious to Clive that Gareth 'knew what he was talking about, knew what he wanted, and was going to get it'. Then Gareth visited Clive to explain his progress so far and the plans he still had in greater detail. A good deal still had to be done but much had already been achieved.

'In the time he had been working on the project he had sorted out setting up a trust fund, becoming a registered charity, as well as a limited company, and he was having talks with Buckingham

Palace about the Duchess of York becoming a patron. He also had the use of big advertising agencies, PR organizations and lawyers to hand . . .' It must have been overwhelming to Clive to realize how little he had achieved by comparison, or indeed how little he knew about what had to be done before his own idea could be a success. 'The ground work they had done was phenomenal. For us to achieve even a fraction of what they had already achieved would have been impossible. They had seen all the major cancer charities and got their support in writing. They had yet to get a TV agreement, so the only ace we had was that we had spoken to Michael Grade . . .' Naturally enough, when Gareth played his trump card and asked Clive to join him in Search 88, saying that his presence 'would be a great asset', Clive had to accept the invitation. He also realized he had no choice.

Nobody seemed to object in principle at first to Clive's continuing to pursue the idea of a Cancer Week, which would now be in association with Search 88, but would still bear his name. With help from others he prepared an optimistic promotional document:

> Clive Jermain's Cancer Week will promote awareness and understanding of the disease and complement Search 88's major fund-raising campaign. The focus of the week will be an exhibition, to be held at a Central London location. The aims of the exhibition are to provide better awareness and understanding of cancer, and it will be a focal point for any interested individual or group . . . this will be the first ever exhibition of its kind – housing under one roof every aspect of cancer research and relief as well as representing voluntary organizations and cancer self-help groups . . . The exhibition will provide a unique focus for a week of television programmes on cancer which will be broadcast by the BBC. Clive has received a commitment from the BBC for this programme activity and he has himself prepared documentaries on cancer that the BBC will produce . . .

Then in his 'thoughts' of 1 May 1987, Clive wrote:

> As I start to type this out I am really straining to keep back

the tears as plans for my Cancer Week have folded ... As I am writing this too I think, why? Why am I writing this down, putting down on paper my personal upsets, failures? Of what interest will my moanings be to anyone else? I suppose that writing it down is a form of therapy ... I suppose, too, that by writing it down I am trying to immortalize my life ... to show people that I did try, am still trying ... I always hoped my play would be successful but the response was really a surprise. All those wonderful letters ... I saw, for the first time, a purpose in my life ... I really praised God and felt so well. People everywhere were talking about it, somebody said that a school was using it in RE lessons and others asked whether there was going to be a book etc. I thought that maybe I might be asked to write the book and I thought that I would be asked to go and talk to different people and groups about it but no, nothing like that. At that time I would have been able to talk about it all over the place, but if I was asked to now it would be very difficult with this new pain, which is constantly gnawing away ... I had never really thought that the play was about 'cancer' but it evoked a lot of interest ... I wanted to do something. I wanted to raise money, but more ... do something more. I came up with the idea for a 'Cancer Week' ... a real piece of immortality ...

The idea was finally killed when Clive received a letter from the BBC informing him that the Corporation's commitment to the many events proposed by Search 88, planned for May 1988, meant that it could not commit itself to what was described as a 'similar event' (which was Clive's week) in 1987. Clive had been very effectively – though not maliciously – elbowed out and he knew that he was powerless to protest. Another 'real piece of immortality' had been scotched. In his dejection he put most of the blame on himself: 'A lot of it was my fault ... there was so much I put off, simply because I was frightened of *people*. I put so many things off and by not pursuing things let others get ahead and succeed.' He allowed himself a degree of bitterness, considering the letter from the BBC to be 'condescending', and wrote in his 'thoughts':

I feel that I failed, but I did try. The opposition, I believe, was not better, but had the financial backing, which made it stronger. I really envy people like Richard Branson, who can come up with an idea and then just carry it out. There are so many things I would love to do, but they are all held back by money and the most frustrating and annoying thing is that the longer and longer I wait the more and more I deteriorate. I do try so hard, but just seem to get nowhere. It makes me wonder how anything ever happens. The most annoying thing, too, is waiting and waiting, then suddenly seeing an idea I had suddenly there, happening. How?

Shortly before the demise of *his* week, the BBC broadcast its own Aids Week. Clive would never have denied the importance and necessity of such a venture at such a time, but it was nonetheless galling for him to have to accept the idea of a television 'week' dedicated to an illness as deadly as his own, but not his own – and without his name on it. There is no denying, either, that the concept of a week of programmes about cancer, with or without the accompanying fund-raising jamboree, was a very good one, especially if it had been handled responsibly and informatively. It would indeed have promoted the 'understanding' that Clive wanted. His idea for a series of considered and enlightening documentaries about cancer – studying the precise nature of the disease, what cancer actually *is*, its history through the ages, its many manifestations and treatments, how it can be halted, how it is controlled when it cannot be halted, the many suggested 'alternative' remedies, the hospice movement, and so on – was an exceptionally good idea. Cancer is an illness about which the majority still knows so very little. Clive understood this all too well and it took considerable courage and will on his part to examine his own ailment in such detail in order to promote greater knowledge.

Possibly a major series will one day be made about cancer, something which pulls no punches, as Clive intended. A good concept always comes to fruition eventually. It is more than likely that it will not have Clive's name on it when it happens, although it would be a fine memorial, far more important than his play. Perhaps as yet the taboo is too strong for a television company to commit itself to such extended coverage of something that too many people still cannot bring themselves to discuss or even think about. Is it significant in any way that the televised 'events' set by Search 88 for May 1988 never materialized either?

Clive continued his association with Search 88, in spite of his sadness at what he called the 'killing off' of his own Cancer Week. Gareth Pyne-James was fond of referring to Clive as his 'inspiration', and Clive, understandably flattered, became fairly convinced for a while that he was not only Gareth's inspiration, but the driving force behind the whole venture. He was never told this in so many words, but he needed to believe it. At times he could be forgiven for assuming it. In the summer of 1987, for instance, a pop song was recorded and released in his honour. Called 'Hold On' and sub-titled 'Clive's Song', it contained a few lyrics which he had written himself. It was extremely soupy and loud. When it was sung on television, a small 'insert' of Clive's face would appear in the top right-hand corner of the screen. It was not very successful, possibly because it was not well promoted, or possibly because of its subject-matter, but probably because it was not a particularly good song. Clive himself, pleased to be its subject, did not know what to think of it objectively. His mother liked it, because it was immediately potent in a way, and it was about her son, which is why she had it played at his funeral. Many other people *pretended* to like it. It was not Clive's finest memorial.

The song was given its first live airing at an enormous Search 88 reception at the Dorchester Hotel in Park Lane, in the presence of the Trust's patron the Duchess of York. The main purpose of the evening was not the song however, but the launch of a book that was to be called *One Day for Life* and which was to contain photographs taken by the general public on a specific day in August 1987. The proceeds were to go to Search 88 and Clive was strongly involved in the book's promotion. In connection with it, and his song, he appeared on the *Wogan* programme, thus making himself known to several million more television viewers.

Terry Wogan asked Clive what some considered to be a highly insensitive question: 'Four years ago you were given a year to live, so what are you doing still hanging around?' Clive himself was not offended by the question. There was a combination of bluntness and humour in it which he appreciated. He was also pleased with it because he was able to quip back: 'Because I've been waiting to appear on your show, Terry.' There was an irony in his reply that the public could not appreciate. Over a year previously, before the transmission of his play, I had endeavoured to arrange for him to be a guest on *Wogan*, but I did not succeed. In any case, if he had been allowed to appear then, he would almost certainly not have seemed so assured as he did now, the seasoned television interviewee. He was in his element and his favourite environment, and he was wholly confident and sharp.

Clive's appearance on *Wogan* provoked further publicity for the book, and a massive response to the request for photographs to be taken up and down the country on 14 August and to be submitted for inclusion in *One Day for Life*. Terry Wogan himself took a picture of his audience on that day. Clive took one of his 'friends at the BBC' in the forecourt of the BBC Television Centre. Both photographs were included in the book, which was undoubtedly Search 88's greatest success. Published in good time for pre-Christmas sales in November, it topped the best-seller lists for several weeks. It was in fact a beautifully produced book and a fascinating record of a nation's life. In an afterword, Richard Hambro, the President of Search 88, mentioned two people who in his opinion deserved special gratitude for the book and the campaign – the Duchess of York and Clive.

'Sometimes,' Clive told me, 'I felt I wasn't much more than a figurehead, or a mascot, and other times I felt I was an embarrassment.' There was possibly resentment in this remark which made it a touch unfair – but it must be remembered that it came from a young man who had wanted to be the active centre of some form of continuous effort which would bear his name, and thus immortalize him, and not merely one of the many participants in a major charitable venture.

He was given a desk and a telephone at the Search 88 offices in Soho Square and for a time he 'went into work' a few days a week. He could not find much to do once he was there. Perhaps this is what caused the 'embarrassment' that he sensed. The sad fact is that he *was* useful to the Trust as someone who could drum up publicity by attracting press attention, or by appearing on *Wogan*. What he was *not* very useful as was as a Search 88 'worker', as one of the faceless and selfless but vital toilers behind the scenes. He was becoming too ill at this time to 'toil' very hard, but he could never have been happy with such a function anyway. The idea of being 'faceless' was anathema to him. Clive was the sort of person who could sometimes feel ignored if the spotlight was off him for the briefest of moments. It was not an especially pleasant aspect of his nature, it has to be said, but it was a cardinal part of his ambition and his achievement. Sometimes it made him seem petty – complaining that his name was not on the sleeve of the record, for instance, although the record itself was at least partly entitled 'Clive's Song', or about being left off guest-lists or out of line-ups.

In the whole business, of course, there were egos as strong as his fighting for attention, and in Clive's world there was only really room for one ego. According to his friend Fiona, Clive's interest in Search 88 was never as intense as it was in the ventures in which he participated more actively and visibly: 'He had to be involved in a much bigger way than Search 88 allowed him to be. He certainly was hurt by the way they seemed to ignore him a lot of the time, for whatever reason they did it. The Search 88 things didn't involve him as much as the play, or *One in Four*. He wanted to be up on the screen, he wanted to be up there with everyone else.'

One in Four is a monthly BBC television programme about disability, and Clive was one of its presenters for five episodes. Its producer, Chris Hutchins, readily admitted to me that he too considered Clive to be at his happiest when appearing on television, in whatever capacity: 'People said that he wasn't allowed to talk properly about his condition on the Wogan show or whatever, but that didn't matter much to Clive, I don't think. What mattered was that he was on television, and to him that was much better than watching someone else on television.'

Clive's involvement in *One in Four*, satisfying to his vanity although it no doubt was, did not arise solely out of the desire to appear on the small screen at any price. He was, at the same time as participating in Search 88, and after the collapse of his Cancer Week, becoming for the first time seriously interested in the problems of disability in society, realizing with increasing sobriety, and as he had never considered in any depth before, that he was a member of a 'marginalized' section of the community, which shared many difficulties unknown to or unappreciated by the able-bodied, and which was clearly discriminated against. Quite simply he began to feel for the concerns of other disabled people. This was a genuine interest, born out of the 'sense of purpose' that to begin with had concentrated on cancer. At conferences on disability he participated with eloquence and he met and discussed problems with other disabled people, many of them quite militant. Had he lived longer than he did, and been able to keep up the energy required, there is every possibility that he might have become quite politicized on behalf of his fellow-disabled.

It was his treatment for a documentary on *Disability and the Media* – the one which began with Clive reading the news in his wheelchair – that first brought him to the attention of Chris Hutchins, but Chris was soon to be impressed by a flood of fine ideas that were not immediately concerned with television or the media in general, but with a whole host of problems of a more personal kind. Clive wanted to do items on the matter of Community Service Volunteers, the 'carers' who provide domestic help for the disabled (a subject close to Clive's heart, for he had experienced difficulties with some of the CSVs supplied to him), or on whether or not the emotional needs of the recently disabled were adequately understood by those treating them, or on the topic of faith-healing, an issue which fascinated Clive more and more the closer he came to death, although he always remained sceptical. Many of the ideas Clive came up with were in the process of being developed when he died. As for his manner as a presenter, Chris understood at once that he had a 'born communicator', a 'natural', on his hands, someone who could simply 'switch it on' for the camera. He acknowledged that Clive may have felt somewhat frustrated by the inevitable 'minority' status of the programme, with its comparatively minuscule viewing figures: 'He wanted to make it in mainstream television, he wanted to be the first disabled newsreader.'

By the time Clive was appearing on *One in Four*, though, or at least in the final programmes he made in the last months of his life, he was resigning himself to the fact that he was not going to 'make it in mainstream television' after all, and that he would have to be satisfied with what he had achieved thus far – too little in his terms, but enough to be proud of. In fact from the time of his first coma in September 1987, silently admitting to himself that death was close, he had to devote his rapidly decreasing energies to matters on the domestic and personal front – preparing himself for the end. Not for the first time in his life, seeing the true balance of things – what mattered and what did not – ambition and fame became what least concerned him. As the Keats poem he was so fond of says, when death is close, thoughts of fame 'sink . . . to nothingness', in spite of Clive's so-often-expressed wish 'to be remembered'.

Even at his most ill, however, he could not entirely reject the concept of exposure before the glare of the cameras, so much did it matter to him, so voraciously had he dedicated his existence to the achievement of that very basic wish. He was still presenting *One in Four*, precariously and often to the concern of his co-presenters, a few weeks before he died. He had also appeared on *Wogan* again, in a Christmas special, and had been a participant in the *Children in Need* 'telethon', when terribly ill in both cases. There was something extraordinarily child-like about his craving to be a part of the television phenomenon to the very end.

Sometimes he wanted what was almost pathetically simple in order to feel satisfaction. Chris Hutchins remembers Clive's 'last request' to him: 'I went to visit him and we were talking about the programme that was coming up, which was actually going to be recorded not far from him, in Dulwich, in one of the other presenters' houses, so there wouldn't be any problem in getting him there and back if he felt he could just make it to the recording, and I told him the sort of things we'd be doing on the programme; for instance, he'd instigated a photographic competition, and I told him that I'd had some entries in and I was going to bring them round so he could start looking at them and decide which ones we should use, and I was just about to go when he said to me, "There's one thing I want to do in the next programme, and that's to read the programme address at the end, I really want to read the programme address on air.'' To want such a very small thing, so very easily obtained, after a short life of wanting the moon, was a humbling desire, and indicative of a kind of perfect, never lost, and finally redeeming innocence. He never did read the programme address on air. A fortnight after having asked if he could – such a tiny request – he was dead.

5

LOVE

I described Clive's play as being among other things 'a cry for love'. In a sense that is what his whole life was – a sustained appeal for affection and attention, which arose from a childhood that seemed to him to contain not enough of either, at least from those that mattered to him most. This was how the psychiatrists interpreted his screams of pain when no other cause of the symptom could be discovered for such a long while. Peter Wells, the priest whom Clive befriended and confessed a great deal to, and who conducted his funeral, told me that he thought Clive's life certainly spoke of great achievement under huge odds, but also of 'unfulfilled love'. More specifically his play, of all Clive's attainments, was the most obvious appeal to one person – his father – to accept him and love him. In the play, Robert's father is not Clive's father – just as the play overall is not in any but the most loose sense autobiographical – but he is nonetheless a man who cannot accept that his son is wheelchair-bound and about to die. He barely speaks to the boy as a result. When forced by his other son to face up to the situation, he declares his love for his dying son in his own taciturn and indirect fashion by suggesting a holiday abroad for the three of them, but Robert dies before it can be arranged. In his first draft of the play, Clive made the father declare his love openly and in so many words: 'I do love you, son.' We thought that such a sudden and direct statement seemed unreal coming from such a man. Clive conceded our point at the time, but got his own back in the stage version of the play a year and a half later when he reinstated the line.

The morning after his play was first broadcast Clive received a telephone call from his father, whom he had not seen for over two years. There were a few minutes of faltering and inconsequential small-talk, although Clive's father did admit to having enjoyed the piece. After Clive had suffered his first coma, six months before he died, he had another telephone call from his father, in which the father said that he would call round to see him soon, but he never did. Such a failure to meet seems all the stranger and sadder for the fact that father and son were not separated by some intractable or even faintly inconvenient distance – the garage in which Clive's father worked was only half a mile or so from Clive's Peckham flat. The gulf was emotional and psychological, and Clive knew the reason. He said to his good friend Elaine not long before he died: 'I can forgive him, you know, it's just that he can't face up to me dying.'

Clive's mother Maureen (Mo to all who knew her well) found Clive's father highly appealing and somewhat exotic when she first met him. Frank Jermain was in his late thirties and divorced, and Mo was eighteen. 'I was young and stupid,' she said, 'and I thought I was in love.' She was, she admitted, 'looking for a father-figure'. Her own father provided her with little or no affection: 'He was a drinker. He used to come home drunk and knock my mum about. I used to climb out of the bedroom window and run away. The police got me and I went to juvenile court but I ran away again. Then I was put in a convent, and stayed there about a year. When I left that I went with the first person that came along just to get away from home.'

Frank was a car mechanic then based in Tunbridge Wells, which is where Clive was born in August 1965. Frank and Mo were not husband and wife at the time but they married some months later. It was a rocky marriage from the start. The rows were not loud, according to Mo, but there was a lot of fuming and steely silence: 'We didn't shout at each other because Frank wasn't like that. He was the type that didn't argue. He'd sooner walk out.' Clive himself recalled the ructions somewhat differently, talking of 'rows and arguments and sitting on the stairs watching them going on'. He also remembered his mother 'walking out a lot', which he could not understand and which for many years he found hard to forgive, considering his father to be the victim rather than the perpetrator. The first serious walk-out occurred when Clive was two. The product of Frank and Maureen's reconciliation after this was Clive's brother Lee. Maureen left again when Clive was five and Lee was three. By then the family was based just outside Heathrow Airport. On both these walk-outs Maureen went to stay with her parents. There was another truce and the family moved to a new home in Chadwell Heath in Essex.

The house at Chadwell Heath was substantial, with a big garden. Clive remembered it as 'the house that was never finished'. Lee recalled: 'Even when we left there wasn't a carpet in the sitting-room. We weren't poor but if you'd come to the house you'd have thought we were poor.' Clive's predominant memory of the place was of being 'left alone with Lee in the big house, or in the garden'. 'We had a shed out the back,' Lee remembered. 'We'd change it into different things every weekend, getting stuff from Oxfam, we turned it into a ship one weekend. We had a swing made out of an old tyre.' Clive described his early childhood to me as 'a happy one which only *seemed* happy because it wasn't really'. The illusory nature of this happiness was based, he admitted, on the fact that 'My brother and I were allowed to do pretty well what we liked all the time because although we didn't really know it then my parents were splitting up.'

There is no disputing that Clive's father was materially generous, described by Mo as 'a great provider' if nothing else, who would ensure that his dependants 'never went without'. 'Even though he wasn't there half the time,' said Lee, 'we'd never go without what we wanted. He wasn't tight by a long shot.' Much of life in the loosely-knit family, however, seemed to be lived on the 'never-never'. Mo could express gratitude for this but also criticism: 'I never worked when the kids were little. My kids had lovely clothes and I had a lovely home – even if half of it wasn't paid for.' Frank always had cash in his pocket. His generosity and fast spending clearly made him attractive to begin with – 'When you're young and thick and in love all that kind of thing is lovely,' said Mo, 'but when you're older and wiser and the bailiffs start knocking on the door you get a bit fed up.' What Frank could not handle at all, it seemed, was responsibility, the very basic business of ensuring his family's continued comforts. Lee at least has learnt a salutary lesson by choosing not to live according to his father's example. 'Money isn't the answer to everything and it's good to have a nice roof over your head.'

In later years Frank would frequently offer Clive the somewhat hackneyed line, 'I've always tried to give you everything I never had as a kid.' He probably meant it, and Clive would reflect that 'maybe it was his way of saying that he loved me'. It manifested itself in Clive's childhood as a constant flow of presents which, like any child, he rather enjoyed receiving – only understanding much later that the lavishing of gifts can be no substitute for true affection. He was, he freely confessed, 'thoroughly spoilt' as a child, materially at least, and without question the favoured son in his father's eyes. The preference was reciprocated – in fact there was an uncomplicated separation of loyalties that split the little family down the middle, Clive siding blatantly with the father, and Lee with the mother, from a very early stage. But Clive was already being offered affection, and in some profusion, from another quarter outside the immediate family. His grandparents – Maureen's mother and father, to whom she kept escaping from her marriage – would insist on seeing Clive at least once a week. 'Every weekend I'd take him to see them in Peckham. If any weekend I said I wasn't coming my mum would cry her eyes out.'

Clive became his grandparents' obsession almost from the moment he was born. The reason for this was very simple – he reminded them of their son, Mo's brother, who had died tragically of a brain haemorrhage when he was only twelve. 'We were on holiday in Wales. He just didn't feel well one day and the same day he was dead. Clive looked just like him.' If Clive was being materially spoilt by his father, he was being even more and in every way spoilt by his grandfather and grandmother, particularly the latter. 'He was allowed to do anything,' said Mo, 'and Lee felt very left out.' Even then she sensed it was not healthy: 'I remember having rows with them about it. And I remember my dad swiping me round the face and knocking me up the passage because I smacked Clive's leg once, when he was about five.'

LOVE

The marriage between Frank and Maureen broke down irretrievably when Clive was seven, shortly after his accident and the onset of the excruciating pain in the back of his neck. Mo went to live with her parents again, and for a while Frank kept the children. Forgivingly Maureen did not interpret this in retrospect as an act of spite, but as the conduct of a father with one unsuccessful marriage behind him already, and four children by that marriage whom he clearly felt he had failed. Clive of course did not mind being left in his father's care, but Lee was enormously upset at being separated from his mother. Frank soon let Lee go. Not much later he had to let Clive go too, because the house in Chadwell Heath had been sold and he had nowhere permanent to live. Clive joined his mother and brother at his grandparents' small 'prefab' in Peckham, something of an indignity after a three-bedroomed house with a large garden in Essex. Mo and Lee moved out of the prefab after about a year, and Clive stayed on with his grandparents. It was the start of a long period of distance between mother and son, and between brother and brother, although contact would always be made at weekends, since no party lived very far from any other.

Frank then reasserted his sway over Clive by sending him to a private boarding school at Reigate in Surrey, for what Mo kindly considered on reflection to be a fine reason: 'I think he thought the world of Clive and he wanted him to have the best education because he saw he was a bright intelligent kid and I think he saw him going places, even then.' Clive interpreted his father's decision to give him 'a good start in life' as being at least partially motivated by a concern on Frank's part for what he already saw as his mother-in-law's smothering and potentially hampering influence over his son. In fact, according to Clive, Frank said as much: 'He accused her of molly-coddling me and said he was sending me away to school to make me more independent.' Clive remembered behaving in a typically inflammable and spoilt fashion after hearing his father say this: 'I ran into the bedroom and I got hold of one of the most expensive things he'd given me – it was a watch – and I stamped on it and smashed it.' Frank's purpose was not vindictive, but actually rather prescient, although Clive at the time could not see it as such. A clandestine, and rather enjoyable, contact was retained between grandson and grandmother: 'She used to send me secret letters, and food parcels, which weren't allowed, so they were always confiscated.'

In spite of the separation from his 'nan', Clive's boarding days were largely happy ones. 'It was a good school academically and the masters were good.' Not that Clive was in any way a notably bookish boy. English was undoubtedly his best subject, but his interests from the very beginning were less literary than visual – making films, of course, editing colourful, picture-filled magazines. He could be grateful to his father in later years for the opportunities the school had provided: 'Looking back I suppose it was the best thing that could have happened. It did in a way set me up for life.' He was not at all interested in playing sport, but he remembered from the start that he liked to *watch* sport – imagining covering the action with cameras, as if he was directing a sports programme for television. He used to do much the same with services in the school chapel. But the most extraordinary legacy that Clive obtained from this school was his accent, which he retained for the remainder of his life and which always seemed surprising when heard in the company of his family, who speak in unmistakable and genuine South London tones. Clive's was a cultivated 'posh' accent by contrast, and it never seemed entirely real – the non-accent of education.

In the battle for Clive's welfare – and heart – between grandmother and father, the grandmother, who was in any case by far the stronger combatant, eventually and inevitably won. Clive recalled how both his father and grandmother turned up at his school one Sunday – his father had broken his arm at work and had had to ask her to drive him to the school – and how from then on she had visited him regularly, or he had been permitted to stay with her at the prefab for the occasional weekend. It was the beginning of a shift of moral and emotional responsibility for the boy that by the time he was thirteen (and regularly hospitalized now because of his scoliosis) was total. Frank did not stop shouldering the financial responsibility, for the straight- forward dispensation of cash had never been a problem to him, and to be fair, he also continued to take an interest in, and often demonstrate an active and impassioned concern for, his son's medical state. Clive's grandfather died when Clive was eleven, thus leaving the boy with the one person in the world to whom he was by now unquestioningly and fawningly devoted – his 'nan'.

At thirteen Clive had to leave the school in Reigate and, because he was hospitalized during the time of the common entrance examination, which might have ensured him a place at a reputable public school, he had to go to a school which would accept him on the basis of its own internal examination. The school was in Blackheath and he 'hated' it, recalling that it had been 'only chosen in desperation really'. He called it 'sporty and uncultured', he was bullied there until he found he could use his medical circumstances as protection, and he begged his father and his grandmother to take him away, within weeks of having arrived. They did not go that far, but they allowed him to be a day boy, and so he spent his nights, weekends and holidays with his 'nan' in Peckham, which contented him. He soon began to spend very little time at school anyway, because of the deterioration of his health. Circumstance was beginning to limit his experience and to narrow his horizons at a time when he should have been opening himself up to all the possibilities – and attendant anxieties – of youth. As it was he was spending most of his time, when he was not in hospital, in a small 'prefab' with an old woman who doted on him – and he was apparently happy to be doing so. When he was fifteen, sudden paralysis cruelly restricted any further experience of life at its fullest in any case.

Even if he had been an entirely healthy teenager, Clive would have needed some persuading to move out of what he knew and felt immediately comfortable with. He was never a mixer, and was very shy. Elaine, who first met him when he was twelve and she was a fourteen-year-old 'Saturday girl' at the local bakery, said she remembered 'this little figure standing in the shop doorway, in his maroon school jacket, who wouldn't come in he was so shy'. He was with his grandmother, and the two of them were already establishing something of a reputation in the area as rather an 'odd couple', the old lady and the small thin boy with the 'posh' accent, which Elaine certainly found strange when he did at last come into the shop and speak to her – after several visits of just standing outside the shop door. When she knew him better, she used to jibe him about his 'posh' voice, and he would reply sharply: 'I do not speak "posh", I just speak slowly.' It was only when his grandmother announced one day that he was 'about to go into hospital for an operation on his back' that Elaine knew he was not well. When he returned from hospital, she started to visit him at the prefab and the visits soon became a regular Sunday afternoon occurrence. Even then, it took a while to get to know the boy well – 'He was very reserved.'

Elaine recollected Clive's grandmother coming into the local bakery – which was, as it still is, something of a social centre in that particular area of south-east London – fairly often, even without Clive, not really to buy much, but 'just to chat'. Very probably, Elaine concluded, she was 'quite a lonely woman' who, since her husband died, 'only had Clive'. Other recollections of Clive's grandmother vary somewhat. Some remember her as a quiet, self-effacing, possibly shy, woman, others as someone who was extremely voluble and forthright. Elaine herself remembered her as 'abrupt'. Peter Wells considered her 'always friendly, charming and polite'. It seemed to depend on what kind of impression she was trying to make, and upon whom, and if she was bothering to make an impression at all. If the television professionals she encountered through Clive found her 'quiet and sweet' on the whole, that was because, according to her other grandson Lee, she was 'putting on her airs and graces'. With those she knew, and on her own patch, she could be extremely talkative – 'moaning usually' said Lee – and very much the centre of attention. Lee's favourite word to describe her was 'strong' – she was 'a strong woman, strong and big'.

She worked until Clive was thirteen, for a banana warehouse off the Old Kent Road 'doing the books', according to Maureen, who also worked there for a while, 'and cutting and packing the bananas'. She seemed to possess prodigious energy, taking her car on excursions, usually with Clive in the back ('Under duress,' Clive remembered, 'I was a stay-at-home') – often to Wales, which was where she came from and where most of her relatives still lived. But by 'strong' Lee also meant strong-minded and opinionated. Her views were rigid, unchangeable. If she took against someone, and she would form an opinion quickly, nothing could be done or said to persuade her that she was wrong, and she would also, as Lee recalled, 'make it clear' to the person in question what she thought, usually by being 'cold, never rude, but you'd know if she didn't like you'. She did not much like Lee, for instance, for the very simple reason that he was not Clive – 'And she could never forgive me for having my health when Clive didn't have his.' Maureen recollected this too: 'Lee didn't stand a chance with my mum. He was always left out.' Without bitterness, Lee remembered that he was always 'the one who couldn't do anything right, and my brother was the one who couldn't do anything wrong'.

All who knew Clive's grandmother agree that she was imbued with a stringent, unflinching puritanism that had a considerable effect on her cosseted grandson. It was most definitely under her influence that Clive wrote to so many television companies with two motives – first, to draw attention to himself, and second, to complain about the bad language in television programmes. Dick Sharples told me how she 'always used to take the *Sun* for the racing fixtures but she always used to remove Page Three just in case Clive saw it'. He described her as 'fiercely protective and very prudish'. She was also a snob, who was very proud indeed when her favourite boy went to a private school and came back with a cut-glass accent. She was highly distrustful of all local people unless she knew them very well: 'She kept herself to herself,' said Lee, 'she didn't like strangers, she didn't make friends easily. Every night at seven she'd shut the curtains, stop the neighbours looking in, that was her attitude to everything.' She was therefore most concerned that Clive should be protected, kept at home, and not be allowed to mix with the locals – young people of his own age and, despite his accent, class. The friends he had made at school were acceptable company, 'the right kind of people', the local youths were not. 'When I used to go down and see him on Saturdays I wasn't allowed to take him over to the park,' said Lee. '*I* could go, on my own, but Clive couldn't.'

Of course it was not just protective snobbishness that made her prevent Clive from 'mixing', and kept him a virtual, though not wholly unwilling, prisoner in her prefab, it was also a terrible fear of losing the only joy she had. 'After my dad died,' said Mo, 'and after she gave up work, what else did she have to live for, except Clive?' She was clearly frightened that if she let him out of her sight for a moment, someone would snatch him away. And thus it was that, according to Mo, 'She didn't let him go anywhere, she didn't let him have a party, she didn't let people come round, she didn't let him have any money. She didn't let him try to do anything for himself – he didn't know *how* to do anything for himself, because she did it all for him.'

Such smothering possessiveness at the time earned her her grandson's undying and adoring devotion, and in any case because of his increasing paralysis he was becoming wholly dependent upon whoever was prepared to care for him. Clive's views on his 'nan' could hardly be objective. He would say of her, over and over again, that she was 'simply wonderful' and to me he said that 'she was like the grans that people talk about – you know, going over to gran's place for the weekend and being spoilt'. He also said that 'She was the only one who took my writing seriously.' This was true. Elaine also recalled that 'It was always his nan who said, "Come on, get up, get writing, Clive." ' Clive remembered his nan as being 'warm' – by which he meant literally, physically warm. 'They were always cuddling,' Elaine said. Clive needed such an uncomplicated, fundamental love – to be cuddled, like a small child, even as a fifteen-year-old boy. And going through traumas of a magnitude unknown to most teenagers – coming to terms firstly with paralysis and then with the prospect of imminent death – he needed enormously strong emotional and psychological support, and there is no doubt at all that it was his grandmother, at this stage of his life, who supplied this – 'She always helped me over the bad bits.'

But when pressed to be honest in his memories of his 'nan', Clive would, with reluctance, admit that he had been restricted in his upbringing because of her swamping affection and concern for him. He too confessed to considering her 'very old-fashioned morally', at least in retrospect, and told me how she would say to him: 'You don't want to mix with the kids round here. Stick with your friends at school.' As a result of which, he recalled, 'I didn't mix at all, and now and then I wanted to,' which made the situation 'quite difficult at times'. His inherent shyness and what he called his 'simple fear of people' made him accept the restrictions imposed on him rather more readily than a more outgoing adventurous teenager would have done – but nonetheless he could not entirely suppress a certain very hidden boyish spirit, even if only in his imagination, as he recollected some years later in his 'thoughts':

> Saturday night for me was just the same as any other night except that I didn't have to get up for school the next day. Saturday evening was spent either amusing myself in my bedroom or watching television. We would sometimes for a treat watch the late film but were normally . . . in bed by ten thirty. I . . . remember lying awake hearing gangs of young people, kids my own age, going past outside, laughing, joking . . . I thought of getting dressed . . . climbing out of the window . . . They would probably have . . . beaten me up anyway, thinking I was some sort of 'funny' case. I never wanted to run away, I just wanted . . . some young company . . . have a smoke, a drink, a swear . . . At the same time I loved nan very much and . . . didn't want to hurt her . . .

He also had sexual fantasies, straightforward enough, no different from those of any other young man with increasingly strong physical desires – mildly exceptional only in that they possessed an obvious sense of 'roughness' which was in marked contrast to the reality of his rather prim existence, and were a clear rebellion in his imagination against his grandmother and all she stood for. On a less immediately sexual level, he confessed to a fascination for his father's work-clothes, and would imagine wearing them. Clothes in general were an obsession with Clive – the clothes he was allowed to wear and the ones he really wanted to wear (his scripts would always be annoyingly full of precise details as to what each of his characters was wearing):

> If ever we went out I always had to be smart – shirt, trousers, and I was considered undressed without a tie . . . For me, I'd have liked to have dressed in T-shirt, leather jacket, jeans and trainers . . . Many's the time I wanted to buy myself a pair of

jeans, or choose other clothes, but it was always done for me by my nan ... When I said I wanted a pair of jeans and a leather jacket ... I was patronized ... with comments like: 'What do you want to look like, a hippy?'

He also liked to imagine possessing full football gear and 'In my imagination I'd climb out of the window and just roll about in the mud in the garden, just to get dirty.' Such thoughts were only attempts to be, at least in his imagination, a 'normal boy'. Unfortunately, as the fantasies continued, he would be brought to the abrupt and depressing realization that he 'had never lived the life of a normal boy' and now never would. At the age of fifteen and the onset of paralysis, all the avenues that he might have explored in his pursuit of normality, but which because of a mixture of his grandmother's hold over him and his own fears he had not, were irrevocably closed to him. Elaine remembered a bitterness which took hold of him 'from the operation onwards' and which never fully left him, despite the occasional happy time, until his grandmother died when he was eighteen: 'He was always religious, but he used to say to me "There's no God up there" and he used to cry and say "Why me?"'

Elaine also recalled suicidal moments when he would say 'The number of times I've looked at those tablets, I've wanted to take the whole bottle I've felt so low.' Not long after his eighteenth birthday he telephoned Peter Wells, with whom he was to form a strong friendship and spiritual bond, and told him he was thinking of killing himself. Peter had just started work at a church in New Cross, not far from Peckham, and was staying at the vicarage attached to the church, 'And the telephone rang one evening and there was this fellow saying that he'd rung the Samaritans but they were engaged and he wanted to talk to someone because he was at the end of his tether and he felt like ending it all.' Peter went round at once to the prefab, which he remembered as being 'small and very damp', and there, with his grandmother in another room – to Peter's dismay because he'd rather assumed that this young man who wanted to commit suicide would be alone – Clive quietly explained 'the desperate state of his life, his pain, and how he felt let down by everybody'. He seemed, Peter recalled, 'very bitter'. Clive's brother Lee also remembered a period of 'bitterness' around this time. It was a stage, he said, when Clive could seem 'very touchy'. Some friends from his first school wanted to come and visit him, but he refused them, saying that 'He didn't want them to see him as he was then.'

Towards the end of this time of lowness, which was shortly before his grandmother died, Clive moved out of the prefab and into a newly built council flat not far away, the flat in which he was to live for the rest of his life and in which he died. This move was not an eighteen-year-old boy's sudden bid for freedom, because the plan was that his grandmother, who was hospitalized then, would move in with him when she was better and the two of them would continue to live together. Because of his grandmother's illness it was his mother who helped him to move into his new home but, as Mo recalled, 'I still had to pick my mum up from hospital to have a look at it, and she'd moan and say, "Why have you chosen plain curtains, why couldn't you choose patterned ones?" I was her daughter, wasn't I, I could never do anything right.'

Clive was permitted a degree of freedom that he had never before experienced, in that he helped his mother choose the furniture and decorations for the flat, so that he could to some extent impose his personality and preferences on the place that was after all to become his first proper home. 'It was him living a proper life at last,' said Mo, 'being able to pick and choose, without having everything done for him.' His grandmother, whose health was failing rapidly, did not possess the power to protest strongly or to assert her hold over him any longer. She spent one helpless and weakened Christmas out of hospital at the new flat, then had to go back almost immediately to the Royal Marsden, where the operation was performed that took away her ability to speak and soon after that she was dead – 'She never came out of intensive care,' said Maureen.

When Clive arrived at the Royal Marsden with Maureen after having been told that his grandmother was on the point of dying, they were too late. She had been dead for about an hour. They were asked if they wanted to see her. Mo said she did not, Clive said he did. He recalled: 'I touched her and she was cold, and she'd always been so warm.' When he returned to his mother she expected him to be crying but he was not. She was overwhelmed by mixed feelings, unable to speak, but Clive had no problem in speaking, apparently saying calmly and controlledly to the ward staff: 'Thank you very much for all you've done for my nan.' On their way home Mo was still expecting him to break down in some way, to reveal his sense of loss – 'We were both silent and I thought, "God, that's it now, he'll go to pieces now," but he never did.' Neither did he cry at the funeral, much to the dismay of everyone present. He retained a calm boyish dignity. 'To my knowledge,' said Mo, 'he's never shed a tear over my mum. And to think that he loved her so much, and she loved him so much.' In an interview for the documentary about him, Clive spoke about the morning after his grandmother's death. He was staying with his mother above the pub at which she was working:

> . . . and I remember waking up the next morning and there was brilliant sunshine outside and men from the brewery had come, crates of beer they were delivering and they were singing and it was just such a shock to hear people singing, and thinking, how can you be singing, my nan's just died. And we were all totally devastated yet the outside world was going on as normal. So really it was a realization that once you die, you're nothing really. The world goes on regardless.

Peter Wells, who certainly knew Clive's spiritual 'inner' state very well at this time, said that there can be no question that Clive was indeed 'devastated' by his grandmother's death (Elaine said, 'He always thought that it'd be him that went first'), and possibly it was straightforward shock that prevented him from mourning her passing with any kind of open demonstration of grief (like the wholly unembarrassed displays of grief at his own funeral). Clive felt very guilty on reflection about the fact that he had not been able to cry. But he felt even greater guilt about having to admit to himself that since her death his life had been freer and more fulfilled. According to Elaine, 'He felt guilty about having a happier and better life since she'd gone. He said in his prayers, "Nan, if you're up there, forgive me."'

Maureen said: 'All she had to live for was Clive, and when she died, Clive lived.' Dick Sharples described her death as 'the opening of a door to a new life for Clive'. Lee also recalled a sudden sense of release at this time: 'He started to realize he had everything he'd ever wanted – his own place, the flat was his, there were no memories there, freedom, he was writing, he could meet people, he could have people round.' Lee's own friends – the local youth so disapproved of by his grandmother – would visit Clive in his flat, and Clive, who 'loved the company of young people', would 'laugh and joke, without having to worry about nan having to get to bed'. Lee described Clive's life with his grandmother as 'routine', whereas now 'Every day was suddenly different.' A bond began to form again between brother and brother – 'It was like I had to get to know him all over again.' Lee remembered spending weekends alone with Clive in the flat, and minor mischief was the order of the day, which to someone who had until then led a protected and sinless existence was intensely exciting: 'With me he could get away with anything he wanted to do, because I didn't care, and there were things he could do with me that he couldn't do with anyone else, stupid things, we used to go down the lane – he'd say "Get that, put it on my lap."'

A relationship that had never existed before also began to establish itself, very tentatively at first, between mother and son. It would take a long time, nonetheless, to become the entirely trusting and loving togetherness that it most certainly was by the time Clive died. To begin with, circumstance alone brought them together, and Maureen was not slow in asserting her new authority. Only about two weeks after her mother's death, she had 'a real screaming match' with Clive – 'We really swore at each other.' She felt she had to make it clear fairly quickly to her pampered son that he could no longer be looked after in the way he had been throughout most of his youth, in spite of his disability and general medical situation. 'For the first time in his life he had to take second place sometimes, which was hard for him to accept. He hadn't got someone who could dote on him and wait on him all the time. He thought I didn't understand him because I couldn't spend all my time with him. I had the pub I was trying to run, I was trying to get his flat straight, I had Lee, I had another life.'

After the row, Maureen claimed, 'We became the best of friends,' which was a forgivable exaggeration (for it took them a while longer to become that), but the air was certainly cleared and it cannot have done Clive any harm. What in fact happened at the end of the row was that Maureen walked out of the flat and straight round to Frank, and she said to him, 'You look after your son, I can't.' It was not long after this that Frank did indeed move in to live with Clive. Maureen continued to visit her son daily, 'making him his lunch', while Frank was out working. She too had to work, however, so Clive had to spend long hours on his own.

Father and son lived together for nearly a year, but there was little communication between them. Frank, as Clive remembered, 'was hardly ever there'. Perhaps it was no bad thing that he was put in charge of Clive's welfare at this particular stage in the young man's life, because Clive would not have been able to explore his new-found independence as fully as he did if he had had a concerned parent watching his every move. But he did often feel appallingly lonely:

Caroline, a nurse at Stoke Mandeville . . . just phoned to give me Graham's number and address. Graham was the only friend apart from Caroline that I made at Stoke. He had wrapped himself around a lamp-post and had really messed up his spine . . . He was really good fun and we got on really well. Then *I* was the one up and standing . . . precariously, holding on to his locker with one hand and feeding him sweets with the other . . . I thought, when I got his number, here I am, lonely, no friend, Graham after leaving Stoke might be in the same position. Maybe we could both be friends again. I rang – it was engaged. After several attempts a girl answered. I asked if he was there, she said 'no, I'm sorry, he's down the pub with his mates'. I asked what time he'd be back, she said 'he normally gets back about half past ten'. She asked who was calling but I said I wanted it to be a surprise. He had friends, mates around him. He didn't need me but I needed him . . . Can you imagine what it feels like?

In his aloneness he also reminisced and regretted:

I was fifteen years old, not unattractive, I thought I was quite good-looking. 'Ooh, you'll soon be having all the girls chasing after you,' our neighbour used to say. I knew what I wanted to do in life, what I wanted from life, I wanted to be someone, not just another Joe Bloggs, I had so much ambition and energy, I wanted to make nan proud of me. I look back at myself now, physically and mentally. I loved what I was. I was a young, attractive, strong, highly sexually motivated young man. I imagined a life of growing up, meeting girls, experiencing, sharing sex, going steady, the one night stands, getting a flat, getting a job, becoming A MAN. A HUSBAND? A FATHER? . . . Oh how I wish I had never had that operation. They took my life away. I stopped living.

Stephen Kramer, a young man then working as a 'carer' for the Spinal Injuries Association and brought in to look after Clive two or three months after the death of his grandmother, recalled encountering 'this boy sitting alone in his flat' enduring what Stephen could only conclude was 'a kind of non-existence'. According to Stephen, 'His dad used to give him breakfast in the morning, then go off to work, then someone would come in and give him lunch, usually his mum, then he'd be alone again until the evening sometimes till late.'

It was not long before Stephen decided to take it upon himself, for the noblest of reasons, to give this reserved and inexperienced lad something of a sentimental education. 'I thought if I'd only got a short time to live I'd be out there, enjoying myself, making the most of the time that was left to me.' He began with the simple pleasures, bringing drink and cigarettes into the flat and talking and getting drunk into the small hours. Clive related the story of his life and Stephen listened, simply appalled. 'One evening I asked him if he wanted to come down to the pub, he said no one had ever asked him to do that before.' Once there, Clive asked, 'What can I drink to get really pissed?' and spent the remainder of the evening downing Southern Comforts. 'I wheeled him home singing, he was grabbing on to lamp-posts, fences, falling out of his chair.'

On another evening they went to Soho – 'which hadn't been

cleaned up then' ('The place of curiosity for many years,' wrote Clive excitedly in his 'thoughts'). Unabashed, Stephen pushed Clive through the garish streets – 'His eyes were popping out.' They tried to get into a peep-show, 'But his chair wouldn't fit the booths.' They decided to go to a strip-joint. As these were all in basements at the bottom of narrow spiral staircases there was a problem of access, but eventually they found one in which the manager was prepared to carry Clive's wheelchair down the staircase while Stephen carried Clive. Once installed, they stayed until the place closed at about four in the morning. It was more of a 'bar' than a strip-club – 'The sort where half a lager costs about two pounds fifty, and the barmaids are topless and come up to you and ask if you want to buy them a drink.' One such topless 'barmaid' naturally approached Stephen and Clive, wandering away again when she realized she was not going to get a drink from them, and then, bored because the night was quiet, returning and spending most of the rest of the night conversing with them – 'She made a real effort to get Clive to open up, which he did eventually, although he didn't know where to look at first.'

It was Stephen, too, who accompanied Clive on 'the fulfilment of a lifelong dream', the trip to Los Angeles and Hollywood. They visited all the major studios, on 'VIP tours' arranged by contacts back in England, and Disneyland, where 'for one down payment you can do all the rides you can cram into a day'. Clive took some persuading to go on the first ride, but once bitten with the thrill he had to do them all, even when the clouds broke and it started to rain heavily and everyone else ran for shelter. He was sick once and towards the end of the day he became so excited and forgetful that 'his condom slipped off and he peed himself', which did not matter because by then it was raining and 'we were both soaked through anyway'.

Clive mentioned this day to me as one of the most uncompli- catedly exhilarating of his life, but there was a suggestion of greater excitement still when he told me that he and his companion had 'got lost' one day in downtown Los Angeles and that they had found themselves 'in a black bar'. Clive never provided me with full details of the incident, for still-lingering prudish reasons. Stephen himself was more forthcoming in his recollections. They had been wandering through one of the less salubrious areas of the city, quite deliberately and apparently at Clive's specific request, when they were approached by two understandably curious black men who invited them for a drink in a nearby bar – which was a 'black bar' because they were in an exclusively black area of the city. Stephen recalled initial wariness on the part of those already in the bar, followed by nothing but friendliness, which he admitted may well have been caused by Clive's disabled state. He also said that Clive, after a preliminary bout of silent shyness, not unlike the first response to the topless bar in Soho, had eventually 'opened up', and he recalled looking over from where he was playing pool with the two men who had invited them in and seeing Clive at a table by the bar talking quite animatedly to a 'gorgeous girl' who was responding with equal volubility. The girl was a prostitute, they soon discovered, and Stephen wondered if he might carry Clive's sentimental education to a logical enough end with the girl's help ('I didn't get the feeling she'd have been unwilling') – but they were 'running out of cash'.

Clive returned to England to face frustrations and occasional despair, caused primarily by the inadequacies and incompetence of other people. All who knew Clive agree that whatever profound internal sadnesses he might have been experiencing, because of his illness, and pain, and impending death, he kept them to himself, rarely inflicting them on anyone else. The unhappiness that he demonstrated more openly (but never to anyone not very close to him) was always the result of the frustration of not being able to do things for himself, of being so 'dependent' and having to rely upon the help of others, who so often proved to be unreliable or no help at all. This problem, which could often lead him to give vent to great choking tears of vexation, was especially borne out in the case of several of his 'carers', or CSVs (short for Community Service Volunteers).

Of course there were some carers – like Stephen, who was not in any case a CSV, but a trained helper from the Spinal Injuries Association, and certain others who *were* CSVs – who proved to be competent, diligent and amiable. They would acquit themselves on Clive's behalf well beyond the call of duty and they became deep friends. But a degree of pot luck seemed to rule. It is Clive's mother who speaks most disparagingly of some of those brought in to look after her son. 'Some didn't even know how to boil a kettle,' she said. She remembered CSVs who 'couldn't even boil an egg, didn't even know how to turn the gas on'. She recalled as an example how Clive had complained to her that he would ask a particular carer to fetch him a bowl of water because he was 'ready to do his bottom half'. The carer would return with a bowl of water and nothing else, and would have to be told with teeth-gritting patience to go and fetch the flannel and the soap as well. 'Can you imagine,' said Maureen, 'you're lying there and you can't do anything, and you're having to rely.' This was, she said, the price that Clive had to pay 'for a bit of independence, for wanting to live in a place of his own'. The social workers, for whom Mo has even less time than she has for the CSVs, would tell her that 'If Clive didn't like the situation, he could always move into a home where he could be looked after properly.'

To be fair to the Community Service Volunteers, the job of looking after Clive in his particular circumstances was an enormously demanding one, for which some seemed simply not to be prepared, and because of Clive's frustration at his own incapacity, allied to an innate impatience, he was not the easiest of employers. Also these 'boys', as Maureen called them (and many of them were only that), had to do things, on the whole uncomplainingly, which made them all, even the least adequate, worthy of a degree of respect. Maureen acknowledged that it must have been 'something to have to stomach' when they had to perform what she referred to as 'the grotty stuff', by which she meant the regular task of emptying and cleaning Clive's bowels. They had to give him enemas to force evacuation, and sometimes when that proved ineffective (as it increasingly often did), they had to resort to 'taking it all out manually'.

To Clive himself, the problem of his inability to have any form of control over his bodily functions was a source of great wretchedness. Of course it was an appalling degradation for him, the ultimate indignity – 'To think you've even got to rely on someone to wipe your arse for you, to put it bluntly,' said Mo – but it was not so much the simple humiliation of the business that made him weep with rage, but far more the prodigious amount of time it took to perform what for most of us is such a trifling everyday task. Clive would have his 'toilet days' – three or four a week – when he could make no appointments or commit himself to anything but the job of going to the lavatory, because a day, most of it spent waiting for something to happen, was often how long it took. Sometimes, Maureen recalled, it would take longer: 'He'd have days when nothing happened and he'd have a stomach ache all day so we'd have to try the next day and that would be two days spent trying to go.'

To add to the shame and sense of inadequacy, Clive would on some days give up and get dressed to face the day in spite of not having emptied his bowels successfully, and suddenly, when he was fully dressed, it would 'all come down at about four o'clock in the afternoon'. The last time Clive experienced such an occurrence to a disastrous extent was only a few months before he died. As a promotional exercise for the book *One Day for Life* he had to meet the Duchess of York and 'go through' the photographs that had been selected for inclusion. Clive was late for the meeting, and the delay was blamed on the traffic whereas in fact it was because he had had difficulty in performing the task assigned to the previous day, which had been an unsuccessful 'toilet day'. The problem had still not been resolved, but Clive decided to risk it. Mercifully, what inevitably occurred took place after Clive had met the Duchess and she had left, but when it did happen it was with a vengeance. Clive had to be hurried to a room that had been set aside for him to rest in after the meeting, but as Mo remembered it 'there was no wash basin so we had to use a bottle of Perrier water'. Elaine and Maureen had to clear up the mess and change Clive's clothes – he had brought another pair of trousers 'just in case' – and, as Elaine recalled, 'it was everywhere'. Both women remembered Clive's tearful sense of shame at the time, but by the end of the day he too was laughing at it. He could see the funny side of the way in which his public and private worlds had been brought into headlong collision. He was as aware as anyone of the ironies that lay close to the surface of his everyday existence.

Another disappointment and cause of great distress on Clive's return from America – in many ways a kind of waking up from a good dream – was the behaviour of his father, which reached a particular nadir at this point. Clive discovered that Frank was enjoying the favours of two women, and for a time neither knew of the other's existence. Although Clive's puritan streak – the legacy of his grandmother – disapproved of such deception, he had to respect that it was very much his father's business as to which women he chose to have liaisons with and how many. Clive knew both women – one, whom he had always thought of as his father's regular girlfriend, he rather liked (she typed out the first draft of *The Best Years of Your Life* for him); the other, with whom Frank now confessed to having an affair, he had known for longer ('she lived close to us at Chadwell Heath') and was not at all certain about (she was 'loud and brassy'), but he could be rather amused by her nonetheless. Clive and his brother Lee used to theorize as to how long it would be before the one found out about the other, and the degree of bloodshed there would be when the predictable happened.

The girlfriend that Clive quite liked turned up one day to find his father was not there when he had told her that he could not see her because he was looking after Clive. This was the first that Clive knew of his father's practice of using his son to play the two women in his life off against each other. Naturally Clive's reaction to this discovery was to tell all to the girlfriend who had just arrived. In Clive's recollection, 'She went beserk there and then, ripped the place apart, searched his bedroom, read his diary.' Then she waited for Clive's father to come home. When he did, 'She went for him.' According to Clive blood was indeed spilt, and Lee's girlfriend who was there by now said to the two brothers 'I knew your family had problems but I didn't think they were this bad.' The woman pulled Frank through the flat and out on to the front lawn and started to hit him, screaming abuse – much to the interest of the neighbours. For some reason, Frank was not wearing any shoes, so it was in his socks alone that he ran away from his attacker and out of Clive's life, because Clive never saw him again.

Clive found it hard to forgive his father for many things – what he could only feel was a slow loss of interest the iller he became, and an ensuing lack of support – but what he found most unpardonable, to the very end, was the using of his illness as a kind of card in Frank's game of deceit. Also of course, at the end, Clive could barely excuse his father's effective absence from the last three and a half years of his life, even though the man lived a mere mile or so away. But there comes a time in the separation of two people, however close, when it is too late for reconciliation, without an enormous effort being made and the swallowing of a great deal of pride – and the reason for this is simple, and awful, shame.

With his father gone, Clive would enjoy even greater independence, and also get to know his mother still better. He would have parties, and his sitting-room would often be crammed with friends, of whom, he now realized with assurance and gratitude, he had a fair number. He also enjoyed 'going out' as he had been unable to for such a significant part of his life, for meals with small groups of relatives and friends, over which he would genially preside, or to the theatre or the cinema.

The fact that his play had been read and liked and was probably going to be made, with the accompanying prospect of resultant recognition from a world wider than that of his immediate acquaintance, gave him a degree of self-confidence he had never felt before. 1985, the year which began soon after his father's disappearance and which ended with the commencement of rehearsals for *The Best Years of Your Life*, was remembered by Clive as a 'happy' year, possibly the 'best year' of *his* life, in spite of the anxiety during its course of wondering if the play *would* be made, of his own creative frustrations, of his continued problems with carers, and most particularly in spite of the fact that he very nearly did not see the year's end, for it was in the late autumn of 1985 that he had to endure chemotherapy after being told that if he did not have it he would be lucky to live until Christmas.

The night before his chemotherapy started, Clive wrote an entry in his 'thoughts' that is here quoted almost in its entirety as a testament to his courage and as a reflection of the increasingly important influence that his faith was having upon him:

Today I did not start my treatment, because of having an eighteen hour fluid drip first. Then, tomorrow, I start the chemo.

This morning I went down to the chapel before breakfast with Rosemary, a wonderfully friendly Christian nurse, where we prayed, silently, read a little, then sung together. I felt so much better and returned to the ward in a fantastically positive frame of mind, and along with the marvellous support and friendship of the staff, notably Sue, Gabrielle, June and Jane. In many ways, today has been a beautiful happy one, which I only pray is not the high before the low. Because although I am really very happy, a steroid induced happiness maybe, as tomorrow draws nearer I do fear what effects the treatment might have. I fear the toxic poisons, pouring through my kidneys, the sickness, which I have escaped from for so long, a fact which has been brought audibly home to me by the man in the next room who has been very very sick all day, and even now as I write I can hear him heaving in his room, a nurse rushes out with another full bowl to empty, hurriedly trying to rush back with a clean one, before another stomach spasm of illness regurgitates the realities of his disease. Oh God, please help that not to be me tomorrow. I also fear being drugged out, being more incapable and being bedridden, and, vainly, losing my hair. But it's all a gamble. Isn't life though, so many people have lived it tell me. So many people react so very differently. Who knows, with my faith in God, and my mind concentrating firmly on my writing, in the hope that I shall become someone after I have died, someone who will be remembered, thought of as a good writer, of not just The Best Years of Your Life but of other things, and someone liked, I might not suffer these side effects and may come through unscathed. I do so hope so as there is so much that I want to do and see, especially before Christmas. I want to get everyone who has been special to me this year a special present. I want to write, see my friends for afternoon teas, dinner parties, have my Christmas party, see Barnum, go to several other shows, decorate my flat and organize a real humdinger of a Christmas with all my family and friends. As well as, most importantly, enjoying the real meaning of Christmas, with so much more significance this year, with Christmas Eve Mass at the Marsden, hopefully reading a lesson, and other Christian events . . .

If this is God's will it will be . . .

Amen.

Clive had faced the full and alarming reality of death's closeness for the first time and had clearly been very frightened by it. Dick Sharples, who visited him in hospital at the critical moment of fear, it seems, said: 'He just wasn't prepared for it. By the time he did die he was totally prepared for it, which was marvellous. He needed that extra time. But he wasn't ready for it that first time he realized he didn't have long. He was shaking, poor little lad.' Now he had to face a treatment the horrors of which he knew, having suffered them already two years earlier. He needed to draw on huge reserves of inner stamina to cope with these awesome thoughts and ghastly prospects. His faith provided him with the necessary strength. He had always had a strong faith – so the argument that he found it in order to cope with his circumstances does not apply – but it was only at this outstandingly important time that his faith became the very centre of his emotional life, as it was to remain for the two years and three months that were left to him.

Clive's faith was based on acceptance, typified by the statement 'If this is God's will it will be.' There was nothing weak about his submission to 'God's will', however. It was not some exhausted capitulation to circumstance, but rather a very strong understanding of his state – a realization that what had happened to him had happened and that he could not change it. According to Peter Wells, 'Clive was not trying to live a saintly life, he was simply trying to be appropriate to his situation.' Upon the basis of this understanding, this acceptance, he would try to live as full a life as possible in the time remaining. As Peter Wells put it, 'He accepted the facts, and got on.' Apart from the prodigious efforts he put into his various projects, inspired by the 'sense of purpose' he had discovered after the transmission of his play, he devoted almost as much energy to the simpler though equally important business of enjoying himself. The parties continued without let-up almost to the very end. Whatever the state of his health at any particular time, not one party was cancelled. It would be wrong to imply, though, that Clive lived the last two years of his life on some kind of spiritual 'high'. He could still be very low indeed, in his more private moments, hit by continued bouts of depression, loneliness, and feelings of great inadequacy, bemoaning his lack of achievement:

> Today evokes a tear drop and an upset stirring of the stomach as inside builds up a well of frustrated anger as yet another day passes and nothing . . .
>
> Yesterday I felt so unwell with a very weasy chest, which got progressively worse through the day, because I cannot cough. I tried and tried, straining and straining to try and cough and move the phlegm, but with little success and much pain. As my feeble attempts passed unrewarded the phlegm, at times, nearly succeeded in choking me!
>
> Two thoughts: 'Oh well I suppose it has been some time since I was last ill with something' and 'Goodbye to another week because of ill health'.

With the continued pain and the reminders every day of his deteriorating condition, the remorseless battering inflicted upon him by one infection after the other, it was a wonder that he was capable of a single moment of spiritual contentment:

> You could say that I am clinging on to life with a ferocity that defies description or, at times, reason. I am just recovering from a very very bad urine infection coupled with some bug and am now getting a cold. Together with this ongoing and seemingly never ceasing pain around my side, stomach spasms and suffering such cold I feel so frustrated and upset at not being able to work at anything – all my body wants to do is sleep – it feels as if my body is giving up on me . . . Constantly my heater is on in my bedroom, glowing brightly and pumping warmth into my deflated body. My only comfort, pain-wise, and way of keeping warm is by lying down in the afternoon covered completely from head to toe by a thermal blanket.

But the fact that, in spite of this appalling and even pathetic state, he was still 'clinging to life with . . . ferocity' is extremely important to an understanding of his faith and how it gave him the strength to persevere. He could so easily have put an end to things, and would occasionally speak of his wish to do so. The means were readily to hand. For so much of his life he had seen no purpose in his pain and his general desolation, his existence had seemed unremittingly meaningless and dark, and he had talked of death as 'a welcome release'. Yet he went on. He accepted his situation, unbearable and inexplicable though it often seemed, and he stuck it out. At his funeral, Peter Wells described a night when a 'figure' had come to Clive and asked him if he could conceive of any reason why he 'should not join Him in His Kingdom', and Clive had responded that he could think of no reason at all. His strength that night was the decision to go on when it would have been so much easier to go under. This is why Clive's life was exemplary, in the literal sense of being an example to follow. Peter Wells said: 'He made it abundantly clear that you could continue.'

Clive's faith was also refreshingly uncomplicated. It was in no sense intellectual, and bore the clear stamp of the very direct Godliness of his grandmother from whom he inherited it, who was according to Peter Wells, 'a simple Godly person who would just ask for a prayer and a blessing'. It was an immediate, very human faith. He would think of God, and Christ, and even the Holy Spirit, as personal friends – 'rather like the imaginary friends a child has and talks to,' said Peter Wells – and he would address them as such. Elaine recalled how Clive would say in his prayers such things as 'Oh just a minute God, I haven't finished, just one more thing . . .' Clive's relationship with his God was not unlike that between God and Adam, walking together in the Garden of Eden. As for his conception of the Holy Spirit, it was so personalized that he had managed to grasp the hardest concept in the Christian faith with a kind of dazzling ease. Because of this very straightforward notion of the figures of Christian belief as imaginable, almost solid, entities, he could not doubt their existence. His illness and his pain would sometimes, and all too understandably, make him feel that God was very far away, but however profoundly desolate he felt, he never seriously considered that God might not be there at all. Also, when he was particularly low, he would complain to and remonstrate, Job-like, with God about his circumstances, but significantly he would never blame Him for them. 'Clive's faith was how I would wish all my faith, my own faith, to be,' said Peter Wells, 'a relationship faith, based on a relationship with a God to whom he complained and moaned but did not blame.'

Clive once had the misfortune to employ a carer who believed in spiritual healing and who became obsessed with the idea of 'laying hands' on him in order to 'make him whole'. As well as being quite comical, the episode was a touching demonstration of the nature of Clive's faith in relation to his illness. He telephoned Peter Wells one evening and asked him to come over to the flat as quickly as possible because his minder, behaving as if possessed, was claiming that he had been 'called by the Holy Spirit' and was trying to lay hands on him, to heal him. Peter had to act as something of a referee between a fixated Community Service Volunteer and his powerless and shaken charge. Clive said that he considered himself 'healed' already. He knew that he could never be healed physically but his sense of spiritual health and inner well-being arose from that very knowledge, from the acceptance of his illness, his disability, and the shortness of his life. He may not have been conventionally, corporeally, 'whole', but the physical limitations of his existence seemed so inconsequential now compared to what he felt within himself, which was entirely and more than satisfactorily whole. The carer, failing to grasp Clive's point, could only reiterate that it was 'the task of the Christian faith to be whole and to make whole', to which Peter Wells retorted, quite angrily, 'Clive is more whole than you will ever be or will ever appreciate.'

Towards the end of his life, Clive's favourite word to describe his spiritual state was 'complete'. It was his strong declaration that his being 'incomplete' in the purely physical sense was of no concern to him whatsoever any more (as it had been his concern, and a cause of great anguish, for so much of his life); neither was the fact that his span on earth would be 'incomplete' in the simple sense that it was going to be a short one. 'What's a fulfilled life anyway?' he once said to me, describing how in a far less certain time he had complained to a priest that he felt he had achieved so little, and was depressed that he would not be able to achieve much more because he was going to die soon, which seemed to him then to be very unfair – and the priest had responded that all lives could be said to be unfulfilled, at whatever stage they came to an end, in so far as there was always something more to achieve, so one could die frustrated at seventeen or seventy. What matters about a life is not its length, but how it has been lived. Clive understood this so well when he died.

He also had a feeling of completeness on a more directly personal level. There had been such an angst-ridden lonely loveless wretchedness about so much of his life, particularly in his teenage years, brought upon him by circumstances – by his physical incapacity of course, and the debilitation of his illness, but also by the swampingly over-protective affection of his grandmother, and the *lack* of true love when it mattered from his parents, especially from his father, upon whose true affection he had so mistakenly pinned his hopes when he was very young and knew no better. In the final months he recognized where the love should come from all the time, and accordingly it came, from his mother. 'The last two years they got closer,' said Elaine, 'but it was only after the coma that they got *really* close. It took a lot to get that bond going.' There is no question of the enormous and strong love that mother and son had for each other at the end – a love compared to which all the anxieties, infatuations, sadnesses and longings of Clive's short life became so insignificant, as Clive himself finally recognized. The 'cry for love' had assuredly been answered. 'He could have gone on for months more,' said Maureen, 'I'd have coped with it. I was prepared to stay with him for as long as it took.'

Elaine told me of a night, about two weeks before Clive died, when he had not yet come out of the Royal Marsden, but when he so wanted to go home, during which the two of them had gone down and talked and prayed in the hospital chapel. It is a recollection that should stand on its own, without comment: 'He said: "Tonight's going to be the night. I'm going to go tonight." He'd been coughing up blood, you see . . . He said, "This is going to be the night" and I said, "Are you sure, Clive?" and he said, "I know" . . . and he said, "Please stay with me" . . . and then he said, "Could you take me down to the chapel," and we were down there until about two o'clock in the morning . . . and he still used to worry about me getting up for work, but I said, "Don't worry, Clive" . . . We talked about everything, everything. He just talked, and he cried, and I cried, we just talked for ages about his whole life . . . about Maureen, about how he was glad that they'd got what they'd got now, they'd never had it before, the bond they had, and he said, "Mo never used to tell me she loved me, she used to find it hard" . . . and he said to me, "There's something I've never ever told you," and I said, "What's that Clive?" and he said, "I really really love you" . . . and we sat and cried together and he said, "I know I'm going, Elaine, and I've made a pact with God." He said, "The other night something happened, I can't even tell you what, but it was a light, a bright white light, to tell me I'm ready to go." He said he'd seen something and that's why *I* believe. I was dumbstruck. I was sitting there and I couldn't believe it. And he said, "I'm happy. You might see me in pain here, you're looking at me and you're seeing me in pain, but inside I'm so happy." He said, "I'm so complete." '

On that same night, Clive asked Elaine to write down a list of instructions to be carried out once he was dead. Entitled his 'wishes', they were written down directly by Elaine as follows:

MY WISHES – 15 FEBRUARY 1988 – PRIVATE

1. TELL MO NOT TO WORRY WHEN I'M GONE. I'LL BE COMPLETE. TELL HER I LOVE HER VERY VERY MUCH.
2. SHE MUST GET AWAY ON A HOLIDAY WHEN I'M GONE.
3. TO BE BURIED.
4. HYMNS. GOD MOVES IN MYSTERIOUS WAYS. THE LORD IS MY SHEPHERD.
5. GIVE THE CAT TO FIONA.
6. FOR US ALL TO MAKE THE RIGHT DECISIONS WITHOUT FIGHTING WHEN I'M GONE. NOT TO UPSET MO.

LOVE

7. MO MUST BE INFORMED OF EVERYTHING THAT
IS TO DO WITH MY AFFAIRS.
8. THANKYOU. LOVE YOU VERY MUCH.

Clive died 'complete' and happy. For a young man of twenty-two, whose life had been one of crisis, anticipation, dashed hopes, intense loneliness, crushing frustration, and above all continuous and unimaginable pain, to have died thus was assuredly an enormous – indeed his greatest – achievement.

AFTERWORD

Recently, on a sunny September Sunday, I visited Clive's grave in Honor Oak Cemetery, Peckham, with Maureen, Lee and Elaine. Five months after the funeral it was still no more than an oblong mound of earth but we enlivened it with fresh flowers. At its head a stone commemorated Clive's maternal grandfather, buried eleven years before. There was no memorial to the influential grandmother, although she was cremated at the same cemetery and her ashes had been scattered there. Clive's own headstone was to be erected soon. Maureen had considered its wording carefully:

HERE LIES MY COURAGEOUS SON CLIVE JERMAIN
DIED THE FIRST OF MARCH NINETEEN EIGHTY
EIGHT
AGED TWENTY TWO
HIS LIFE IS OUR MEMORY
HIS ABSENCE OUR SILENT GRIEF
GOODNIGHT MY DARLING NOT FAREWELL
NEVER OUT OF OUR THOUGHTS
TILL WE MEET AGAIN

Maureen tended the grave, as she had done regularly since the funeral, and told me how, when the headstone was in place, she was going to have it properly turfed. Lee and Elaine, chatting and joking, fetched water. I took photographs of the three of them at the graveside. It was not a gloomy visit. We were there at my instigation, to remember 'the good times', the occasions in Clive's life and the aspects of his nature which provoked love and laughter, and which again did so now. These close ones had read the first draft of the book and had expressed concern at its emphasis on the dark side of Clive's story; the least I could do now was to allow them to reiterate the happy and loving moments, of which there had been so many.

We went for Sunday lunch at the Star Café at Peckham Rye, which had been one of Clive's favourite eating places. Elaine, always the garrulous one, had the most to say about the jocular side of Clive's nature. He was a master of the practical joke, and because he was a fine performer, with a host of practised and convincing accents to hand, he could sustain these pretences for a long time. Elaine herself, after knowing him and his ways for many years, could still fall into the trap of believing he was someone else when he telephoned her. He liked pretending to be an anonymous 'secret admirer'. He thrived on harmless embarrassment. Once he subjected Elaine to a diatribe in the back of a taxi, loudly so that the taxi driver could hear every word, about how he was not pleased with her services as an 'escort' and how he would have to ask the escort agency that had provided her to send him someone more attractive and co-operative next time. Typically, his performance did not falter throughout the entire journey.

Maureen spoke mainly of Clive's adroitness as a host, a subject which was taken up by Lee and Elaine. There was never a shortage of true friends to fill his many unstinting and well-organized parties, or the smaller groups he would take out to restaurants, for Clive inspired genuine and immediate fondness in all those who met him. It was rarely, in my experience, an affection that sprang from sympathy, as it could so easily have been in a less inherently charming person. He possessed, to quite an astounding extent, a natural ability to disarm people to such a degree that they forgot his clinical situation and his disability within minutes. He was a fully generous person, with a prodigious generosity of spirit, an exceptional tolerance and understanding, and an almost childlike unwillingness to offend. The possibility of having offended, even in the smallest way, would send him into a spiral of remorse.

Clive was also materially generous (and he never had much money). For this reason – as well as for its relevance to his faith – Christmas was his favourite time of year, because it involved the joy of giving. In the weeks before Christmas, detailed present lists would be made and shopping expeditions into the West End would be organized, the high point of which was an exhausting day at Harrods. I could always expect a Harrods hamper from Clive at Christmas. His parties were a reflection of his selfless munificence too. They were thrown for the pleasure of watching others enjoying themselves. Many who remember Clive remember him best for his parties. Excuses were only rarely proffered; nobody would willingly turn down an invitation, and he knew a lot of very busy people.

He was, as Maureen reminded me on this day when we had gathered to recollect the good times, planning parties almost to the very end. In the last days of his life, when he knew he would soon die and he had so many arrangements to make to ensure a 'good death', one of the several lists he could not avoid making even then was of a small group of friends that he wanted to invite to dinner, 'in case', as Maureen put it, 'a miracle happened'. In the state he was in it would indeed have been a miracle if he had survived yet again, and it was entirely typical of Clive that the way he wanted to celebrate such an improbability was with a joyful gathering, as soon as possible, of those he loved most and who loved him so profoundly. He died with enormous affection in his heart.

FOR THE BEST IN PAPERBACKS, LOOK FOR THE 🐧

In every corner of the world, on every subject under the sun, Penguin represents quality and variety – the very best in publishing today.

For complete information about books available from Penguin – including Puffins, Penguin Classics and Arkana – and how to order them, write to us at the appropriate address below. Please note that for copyright reasons the selection of books varies from country to country.

In the United Kingdom: Please write to *Dept E.P., Penguin Books Ltd, Harmondsworth, Middlesex, UB7 0DA.*

If you have any difficulty in obtaining a title, please send your order with the correct money, plus ten per cent for postage and packaging, to *PO Box No 11, West Drayton, Middlesex*

In the United States: Please write to *Dept BA, Penguin, 299 Murray Hill Parkway, East Rutherford, New Jersey 07073*

In Canada: Please write to *Penguin Books Canada Ltd, 2801 John Street, Markham, Ontario L3R 1B4*

In Australia: Please write to the *Marketing Department, Penguin Books Australia Ltd, P.O. Box 257, Ringwood, Victoria 3134*

In New Zealand: Please write to the *Marketing Department, Penguin Books (NZ) Ltd, Private Bag, Takapuna, Auckland 9*

In India: Please write to *Penguin Overseas Ltd, 706 Eros Apartments, 56 Nehru Place, New Delhi, 110019*

In the Netherlands: Please write to *Penguin Books Netherlands B.V., Postbus 195, NL–1380AD Weesp*

In West Germany: Please write to *Penguin Books Ltd, Friedrichstrasse 10–12, D–6000 Frankfurt/Main 1*

In Spain: Please write to *Longman Penguin España, Calle San Nicolas 15, E–28013 Madrid*

In Italy: Please write to *Penguin Italia s.r.l., Via Como 4, I-20096 Pioltello (Milano)*

In France: Please write to *Penguin Books Ltd, 39 Rue de Montmorency, F-75003 Paris*

In Japan: Please write to *Longman Penguin Japan Co Ltd, Yamaguchi Building, 2–12–9 Kanda Jimbocho, Chiyoda-Ku, Tokyo 101*

FOR THE BEST IN PAPERBACKS, LOOK FOR THE 🐧

PENGUIN HEALTH

Audrey Eyton's F-Plus   Audrey Eyton

'Your short cut to the most sensational diet of the century' – *Daily Express*

Baby and Child   Penelope Leach

A beautifully illustrated and comprehensive handbook on the first five years of life. 'It stands head and shoulders above anything else available at the moment' – Mary Kenny in the *Spectator*

Woman's Experience of Sex   Sheila Kitzinger

Fully illustrated with photographs and line drawings, this book explores the riches of women's sexuality at every stage of life. 'A book which any mother could confidently pass on to her daughter – and her partner too' – *Sunday Times*

Food Additives   Erik Millstone

Eat, drink and be worried? Erik Millstone's hard-hitting book contains powerful evidence about the massive risks being taken with the health of the consumer. It takes the lid off food and the food industry.

Living with Allergies   Dr John McKenzie

At least 20% of the population suffer from an allergic disorder at some point in their lives and this invaluable book provides accurate and up-to-date information about the condition, where to go for help, diagnosis and cure – and what we can do to help ourselves.

Living with Stress   Cary L. Cooper, Rachel D. Cooper and Lynn H. Eaker

Stress leads to more stress, and the authors of this helpful book show why low levels of stress are desirable and how best we can achieve them in today's world. Looking at those most vulnerable, they demonstrate ways of breaking the vicious circle that can ruin lives.

A CHOICE OF PENGUINS

The Russian Album Michael Ignatieff

Michael Ignatieff movingly comes to terms with the meaning of his own family's memories and histories, in a book that is both an extraordinary account of the search for roots and a dramatic and poignant chronicle of four generations of a Russian family.

Beyond the Blue Horizon Alexander Frater

The romance and excitement of the legendary Imperial Airways East-bound Empire service – the world's longest and most adventurous scheduled air route – relived fifty years later in one of the most original travel books of the decade. 'The find of the year' – *Today*

Getting to Know the General Graham Greene

'In August 1981 my bag was packed for my fifth visit to Panama when the news came to me over the telephone of the death of General Omar Torrijos Herrera, my friend and host...' 'Vigorous, deeply felt, at times funny, and for Greene surprisingly frank' – *Sunday Times*

The Search for the Virus Steve Connor and Sharon Kingman

In this gripping book, two leading *New Scientist* journalists tell the remarkable story of how researchers discovered the AIDS virus and examine the links between AIDS and lifestyles. They also look at the progress being made in isolating the virus and finding a cure.

Arabian Sands Wilfred Thesiger

'In the tradition of Burton, Doughty, Lawrence, Philby and Thomas, it is, very likely, the book about Arabia to end all books about Arabia' – *Daily Telegraph*

Adieux: A Farewell to Sartre Simone de Beauvoir

A devastatingly frank account of the last years of Sartre's life, and his death, by the woman who for more than half a century shared that life. 'A true labour of love, there is about it a touching sadness, a mingling of the personal with the impersonal and timeless which Sartre himself would surely have liked and understood' – *Listener*

A CHOICE OF PENGUINS

Trail of Havoc Patrick Marnham

In this brilliant piece of detective work, Patrick Marnham has traced the steps of Lord Lucan from the fateful night of 7 November 1974 when he murdered his children's nanny and attempted to kill his ex-wife. As well as being a fascinating investigation, the book is also a brilliant portrayal of a privileged section of society living under great stress.

Light Years Gary Kinder

Eduard Meier, an uneducated Swiss farmer, claims since 1975 to have had over 100 UFO sightings and encounters with 'beamships' from the Pleiades. His evidence is such that even the most die-hard sceptics have been unable to explain away the phenomenon.

And the Band Played On Politics, People and the AIDS Epidemic
Randy Shilts

Written after years of extensive research by the only American journalist to cover the epidemic full-time, *And the Band Played On* is a masterpiece of reportage and a tragic record of mismanaged institutions and scientific vendettas, of sexual politics and personal suffering.

The Return of a Native Reporter Robert Chesshyre

Robert Chesshyre returned to Britain in 1985 from the United States, where he had spent four years as the *Observer*'s correspondent. This is his devastating account of the country he came home to: intolerant, brutal, grasping and politically and economically divided. It is a nation, he asserts, struggling to find a role.

Women and Love Shere Hite

In this culmination of *The Hite Report* trilogy, 4,500 women provide an eloquent testimony to the disturbingly unsatisfying nature of their emotional relationships and point to what they see as the causes. *Women and Love* reveals a new cultural perspective in formation: as women change the emotional structure of their lives, they are defining a fundamental debate over the future of our society.

FOR THE BEST IN PAPERBACKS, LOOK FOR THE 🐧

A CHOICE OF PENGUINS

The Secret Lives of Trebitsch Lincoln   Bernard Wasserstein

Trebitsch Lincoln was Member of Parliament, international spy, right-wing revolutionary, Buddhist monk – and this century's most extraordinary conman. 'Surely the final work on a truly extraordinary career' – Hugh Trevor-Roper. 'An utterly improbable story ... a biographical coup' – *Guardian*

Out of Africa   Karen Blixen (Isak Dinesen)

After the failure of her coffee-farm in Kenya, where she lived from 1913 to 1931, Karen Blixen went home to Denmark and wrote this unforgettable account of her experiences. 'No reader can put the book down without some share in the author's poignant farewell to her farm' – *Observer*

In My Wildest Dreams   Leslie Thomas

The autobiography of Leslie Thomas, author of *The Magic Army* and *The Dearest and the Best*. From Barnardo boy to original virgin soldier, from apprentice journalist to famous novelist, it is an amazing story. 'Hugely enjoyable' – *Daily Express*

The Winning Streak   Walter Goldsmith and David Clutterbuck

Marks and Spencer, Saatchi and Saatchi, United Biscuits, GEC ... The UK's top companies reveal their formulas for success, in an important and stimulating book that no British manager can afford to ignore.

Bird of Life, Bird of Death   Jonathan Evan Maslow

In the summer of 1983 Jonathan Maslow set out to find the quetzal. In doing so, he placed himself between the natural and unnatural histories of Central America, between the vulnerable magnificence of nature and the terrible destructiveness of man. 'A wonderful book' – *The New York Times Book Review*

Mob Star   Gene Mustain and Jerry Capeci

Handsome, charming, deadly, John Gotti is the real-life Mafia boss at the head of New York's most feared criminal family. *Mob Star* tells the chilling and compelling story of the rise to power of the most powerful criminal in America.

FOR THE BEST IN PAPERBACKS, LOOK FOR THE 🐧

A CHOICE OF PENGUINS

Riding the Iron Rooster Paul Theroux

An eye-opening and entertaining account of travels in old and new China, from the author of *The Great Railway Bazaar*. 'Mr Theroux cannot write badly ... in the course of a year there was almost no train in the vast Chinese rail network on which he did not travel' – Ludovic Kennedy

The Markets of London Alex Forshaw and Theo Bergstrom

From Camden Lock and Columbia Road to Petticoat Lane and Portobello Road, from the world-famous to the well-kept secrets, here is the ultimate guide to London's markets: as old, as entertaining and as diverse as the capital itself.

The Chinese David Bonavia

'I can think of no other work which so urbanely and entertainingly succeeds in introducing the general Western reader to China' – *Sunday Telegraph*. 'Strongly recommended' – *The Times Literary Supplement*

The Diary of Virginia Woolf
Five volumes edited by Quentin Bell and Anne Olivier Bell

'As an account of intellectual and cultural life of our century, Virginia Woolf's diaries are invaluable; as the record of one bruised and unquiet mind, they are unique' – Peter Ackroyd in the *Sunday Times*

Voices of the Old Sea Norman Lewis

'I will wager that *Voices of the Old Sea* will be a classic in the literature about Spain' – *Mail on Sunday*. 'Limpidly and lovingly, Norman Lewis has caught the helpless, unwitting, often foolish, but always hopeful village in its dying summers, and saved the tragedy with sublime comedy' – *Observer*

Ninety-Two Days Evelyn Waugh

With characteristic honesty, Evelyn Waugh here debunks the romantic notions attached to rough travelling. His journey in Guiana and Brazil is difficult, dangerous and extremely uncomfortable, and his account of it is witty and unquestionably compelling.

PENGUIN HEALTH

Living with Asthma and Hay Fever   John Donaldson

For the first time, there are now medicines that can prevent asthma attacks from taking place. Based on up-to-date research, this book shows how the majority of sufferers can beat asthma and hay fever and lead full and active lives.

Anorexia Nervosa   R. L. Palmer

Lucid and sympathetic guidance for those who suffer from this disturbing illness, and for their families and professional helpers, given with a clarity and compassion that will make anorexia more understandable and consequently less frightening for everyone involved.

Medicines: A Guide for Everybody   Peter Parish

This sixth edition of a comprehensive survey of all the medicines available over the counter or on prescription offers clear guidance for the ordinary reader as well as invaluable information for those involved in health care.

Pregnancy and Childbirth   Sheila Kitzinger

A complete and up-to-date guide to physical and emotional preparation for pregnancy – a must for all prospective parents.

The Penguin Encyclopaedia of Nutrition   John Yudkin

This book cuts through all the myths about food and diets to present the real facts clearly and simply. 'Everyone should buy one' – *Nutrition News and Notes*

The Parents' A to Z   Penelope Leach

For anyone with children of 6 months, 6 years or 16 years, this guide to all the little problems involved in their health, growth and happiness will prove reassuring and helpful.

Positive Smear Susan Quilliam

A 'positive' cervical smear result is not only a medical event but an emotional event too: one which means facing up to issues surrounding your sexuality, fertility and mortality. Based on personal experiences, Susan Quilliam's practical guide will help every woman meet that challenge.

Medicine The Self-Help Guide
Professor Michael Orme and Dr Susanna Grahame-Jones

A new kind of home doctor – with an entirely new approach. With a unique emphasis on self-management, *Medicine* takes an *active* approach to drugs, showing how to maximize their benefits, speed up recovery and minimize dosages through self-help and non-drug alternatives.

Defeating Depression Tony Lake

Counselling, medication and the support of friends can all provide invaluable help in relieving depression. But if we are to combat it once and for all we must face up to perhaps painful truths about our past and take the first steps forward that can eventually transform our lives. This lucid and sensitive book shows us how.

Freedom and Choice in Childbirth Sheila Kitzinger

Undogmatic, honest and compassionate, Sheila Kitzinger's book raises searching questions about the kind of care offered to the pregnant woman – and will help her make decisions and communicate effectively about the kind of birth experience she desires.

Care of the Dying Richard Lamerton

It is never true that 'nothing more can be done' for the dying. This book shows us how to face death without pain, with humanity, with dignity and in peace.

Just for William   Nicholas Woolley and Sue Clayton

Originating as a film for the award-winning BBC2 documentary series *Forty Minutes*, *Just for William* is the story of William Clayton, diagnosed with leukaemia at the age of nine – and the story of a family who refused to give up hope in the battle against one of the deadliest diseases of all.

The Secret Lives of Trebitsch Lincoln   Bernard Wasserstein

Trebitsch Lincoln was Member of Parliament, international spy, right-wing revolutionary, Buddhist monk – and this century's most extra-ordinary conman. 'An utterly improbable story … a biographical scoop' – *Guardian*

Tolstoy   A. N. Wilson

'One of the best biographies of our century' – Leon Edel. 'All his skills as a writer, his fire as a critic, his insight as a novelist and his experience of life have come together in this subject' – Peter Levi in the *Independent*

Fox on the Run   Graeme Fowler

The intimate diary of a dramatic eighteen months, in which Fowler became the first Englishman to score a double century in India – before being cast down by injury and forced to come to terms with loss of form. 'One of the finest cricket books this year' – *Yorkshire Post*. Winner of the first Observer/Running Late Sports Book Award.

Backcloth   Dirk Bogarde

The final volume of Dirk Bogarde's autobiography is not about his acting years but about Dirk Bogarde the man and the people and events that have shaped his life and character. All are remembered with affection, nostalgia and characteristic perception and eloquence.

Jackdaw Cake   Norman Lewis

From Carmarthen to Cuba, from Enfield to Algeria, Norman Lewis brilliantly recounts his transformation from stammering schoolboy to the man Auberon Waugh called 'the greatest travel writer alive, if not the greatest since Marco Polo'.